Your *Clinics* subscription just got better!

You can now access the FULL TEXT of this publication online at no additional cost! Activate your online subscription today and receive...

- Full text of all issues from 2002 to the present
- Photographs, tables, illustrations, and references
- Comprehensive search capabilities
- Links to MEDLINE and Elsevier journals

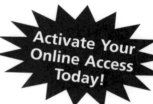

Activate Your Online Access Today!

Plus, you can also sign up for E-alerts of upcoming issues or articles that interest you, and take advantage of exclusive access to bonus features!

To activate your individual online subscription:

1. Visit our website at **www.TheClinics.com**.

2. Click on "Register" at the top of the page, and follow the instructions.

3. To activate your account, you will need your subscriber account number, which you can find on your mailing label (note: the number of digits in your subscriber account number varies from six to ten digits). See the sample below where the subscriber account number has been circled.

This is your subscriber account number

```
****************************
FEB00  J0167  C7

J.H. DOE, MD
531 MAIN ST
CENTER CITY, NY  10001-001
```

D1306983

4. That's it! Your online access to the most trusted source for clinical reviews is now available.

theclinics.com

ELSEVIER

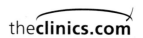

NURSING CLINICS
OF NORTH AMERICA

Wound Care

WITHDRAWN

GUEST EDITOR
Barbara Pieper, PhD, RN, CS, CWOCN, FAAN

June 2005 • Volume 40 • Number 2

SAUNDERS

An Imprint of Elsevier, Inc.
PHILADELPHIA   LONDON   TORONTO   MONTREAL   SYDNEY   TOKYO

W.B. SAUNDERS COMPANY
A Division of Elsevier Inc.

1600 John F. Kennedy Blvd., Suite 1800, Philadelphia, PA 19103-2899.

http://www.theclinics.com

THE NURSING CLINICS OF NORTH AMERICA
June 2005
Editor: Maria Lorusso

Volume 40, Number 2
ISSN 0029-6465
ISBN 1-4160-2737-8

The ideas and opinions expressed in *The Nursing Clinics of North America* do not necessarily reflect those of the Publisher. The Publisher does not assume any responsibility for any injury and/or damage to persons or property arising out of or related to any use of the material contained in this periodical. The reader is advised to check the appropriate medical literature and the product information currently provided by the manufacturer of each drug to be administered to verify the dosage, the method and duration of administration, or contraindications. It is the responsibility of the treating physician or other health care professional, relying on independent experience and knowledge of the patient, to determine drug dosages and the best treatment for the patient. Mention of any product in this issue should not be construed as endorsement by the contributors, editors, or the Publisher of the product or manufacturers' claims.

The Nursing Clinics of North America (ISSN 0029-6465) is published quarterly by Elsevier Inc., Corporate and Editorial Offices: Elsevier Inc., 1600 John F. Kennedy Blvd., Suite 1800, Philadelphia, PA 19103-2899. Accounting and Circulation Offices: 6277 Sea Harbor Drive, Orlando, FL 32887-4800. Periodicals postage paid at Orlando, FL 32862, and additional mailing offices. Subscription price per year is, $100.00 (US individuals), $191.00 (US institutions), $165.00 (international individuals), $225.00 (international institutions), $138.00 (Canadian individuals), $225.00 (Canadian institutions), $55.00 (US students), and $83.00 (international students). To receive student/resident rate, orders must be accompanied by name of affiliated institution, date of term, and the signature of program/residency coordinator on institution letterhead. Orders will be billed at individual rate until proof of status is received. Foreign air speed delivery is included in all *Clinics* subscription prices. All prices are subject to change without notice. POSTMASTER: Send address changes to W.B. Saunders Company, Periodicals Fulfillment, Orlando, FL 32887-4800. **Customer Service: 1-800-654-2452 (US). From outside of the US, call 1-407-345-4000.**

Nursing Clinics of North America is covered in *EMBASE/Excerpta Medica, Index Medicus, Social Sciences Citation Index, Current Contents, ASCA, Cumulative Index to Nursing, RNdex Top 100,* and *Allied Health Literature and International Nursing Index (INI).*

Printed in the United States of America.

GUEST EDITOR

BARBARA PIEPER, PhD, RN, CS, CWOCN, FAAN, Professor, College of Nursing, Wayne State University; and Nurse Practitioner, Detroit Receiving Hospital, Detroit, Michigan

CONTRIBUTORS

JANICE M. BEITZ, PhD, RN, CS, CNOR, CWOCN, Associate Professor; Director of Nursing Certificate and Distributive Learning Programs; and WOCNEP Co-Director, School of Nursing, La Salle University, Philadelphia, Pennsylvania

MARIA HELENA LARCHER CALIRI, PhD, RN, Associate Professor, Ribeirao Preto College of Nursing, University of Sao Paulo; and WHO Collaborating Centre for Nursing Research Development, Ribeirao Preto, Sao Paulo, Brazil

BERNADETTE CULLEN, MSN, RN, CWOCN, Vice President, Acute/Post Acute Nursing Services, East Jefferson General Hospital, Metairie, Louisiana

DOROTHY DOUGHTY, MN, RN, CWOCN, FAAN, Emory University Wound Ostomy Continence Nursing Education Center, Emory University, Atlanta, Georgia

JOHN R. EBRIGHT, MD, Associate Professor, Department of Internal Medicine, Wayne State University School of Medicine; and Division of Infectious Diseases, Harper University Hospital, Detroit, Michigan

SUSAN GALLAGHER, RN, CWOCN, MA, MSN, PhD, Houston, Texas

MARY A. GERLACH, MSN, APRN-BC, CWOCN, Clinical Nurse Specialist, Division of Nursing, St. Joseph's Mercy of Macomb Hospital, Clinton Township, Michigan

HARRIET W. HOPF, MD, Associate Professor, Department of Anesthesiology and Perioperative Care, University of California San Francisco, San Francisco, California

JOHN A. HOPPER, MD, Assistant Professor, Wayne State University School of Medicine, Detroit, Michigan

DIANNE MACKEY, BSN, RN, PHN, CWOCN, Wound/Skin Coordinator, Home Health/Hospice Department, Kaiser Permanente; and Vice President, Wound, Ostomy and Continence Nurses Society, San Diego, California

JOANN MAKLEBUST, MSN, APRN-BC, AOCN, FAAN, Clinical Nurse Specialist/Wound Care, Nurse Practitioner/Oncologic Surgery, Karmanos Cancer Institute, Detroit Medical Center; and Adjunct Associate Clinical Professor, College of Nursing, Wayne State University, Detroit, Michigan

BARBARA PIEPER, PhD, RN, CS, CWOCN, FAAN, Professor, College of Nursing, Wayne State University; and Nurse Practitioner, Detroit Receiving Hospital, Detroit, Michigan

STEPHANIE MYERS SCHIM, PhD, RN, CNAA, APRN, BC, Assistant Professor, College of Nursing, Wayne State University, Detroit, Michigan

MARY SIEGGREEN, MSN, APRN, CVN, Nurse Practitioner, Department of Vascular Surgery, Harper University Hospital, Detroit Medical Center, Detroit, Michigan; and Assistant Clinical Professor, College of Nursing, Wayne State University, Northville, Michigan

NANCY A. STOTTS, RN, EdD, FAAN, Professor, Department of Physiological Nursing, University of California San Francisco, San Francisco, California

JOANNE D. WHITNEY, PhD, RN, CWCN, FAAN, Professor, Biobehavioral Nursing and Health Systems, University of Washington, School of Nursing, Seattle, Washington

CONTRIBUTORS

CONTENTS

Knowledge of normal wound healing and the changes associated with chronic wounds have advanced significantly. Distinct characteristics identified through basic and clinical studies are found in nonhealing wounds, including bacterial and growth factor imbalances, increased inflammatory responses, and proteolytic forces that tip the balance toward tissue degradation rather than repair. This article describes the alterations that reduce healing and that also have important implications for the management of chronic wounds and presents a focus for future developments in wound therapy.

This article discusses the use of topical antimicrobial agents for promoting healing in clinically uninfected wounds. Chronic pressure and leg ulcers are predictably colonized by multiple microorganisms including anaerobic and aerobic bacteria. In most instances, these organisms are clinically irrelevant and do not warrant antibiotic treatment. Topical or systemic antibodies are indicated for the treatment of patients with invasive infection and before ulcer closure, if quantitative tissue culture is positive. However, treating patients with topical antimicrobial agents for clinically uninfected but slowly healing wounds cannot be recommended at this time. Currently, evidence is insufficient to support routine use of antimicrobial agents for this purpose.

FORTHCOMING ISSUES

RECENT ISSUES

ELSEVIER
SAUNDERS

NURSING
CLINICS
OF NORTH AMERICA

Nurs Clin N Am 40 (2005) xi–xiii

Preface

Wound Care

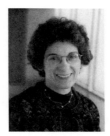

Barbara Pieper, PhD, RN, CS, CWOCN, FAAN
Guest Editor

Wounds and wound care continue to challenge patients, families, professionals, and health care systems. Although prevention is often the goal, all wounds cannot be prevented; and unfortunately, all wounds will not heal. Basic and clinical scientists continue to learn more about the wound process and healing. Microorganisms, including aerobic and anaerobic bacteria, growth factors, the inflammatory response, and proteolytic factors may shift wounds to a nonhealing state. The presence of a wound frequently raises questions about infection and when and how to treat the infection. This issue of *Nursing Clinics of North America* presents an update on the wound process, healing, and intervening factors; discussion includes the impact of microorganisms on chronic pressure ulcers and leg ulcers and when the need arises for antibiotic therapy.

The number of older adults is increasing. Older adults have multiple health care problems, consume multiple medications, and have physiologic changes in wound healing. Older adults may lack transportation for frequent wound care visits and a supportive person in the home to assist with wound care. The majority of older adults will be hospitalized at some point in later life, resulting in a crisis event [1]. Hospitalization increases the person's chance of developing a chronic wound, such as a pressure ulcer. In addition, older adults are undergoing operative procedures. End of life provides additional concerns about balancing patient comfort and wound care goals. This issue shares ideas about wound care for the older adult and at end of life.

Pressure ulcers and lower extremity ulcers are common chronic wounds. Both categories are significant threats to a person's health and well being.

doi:10.1016/j.cnur.2004.09.017

This issue presents updates on pressure ulcers and lower extremity ulcers. Persons at risk or who have pressure or chronic lower extremity ulcers need reinforcement of teaching, strategies for prevention, and assistance with wound care.

Nurses are challenged to realize wound care issues in persons who formerly were not frequently discussed. Bariatrics, or health care for the obese, has evolved from unhealthy lifestyles in the United States, where body weight has increased. Obesity increases concern about the development and treatment of wounds. Furthermore, obese individuals may need specialized equipment (eg, beds, chairs, walkers, and lift devices) to match their body weight and multiple caregivers to provide the care. Large urban centers have an increased frequency of substance abuse (eg, alcohol, cigarettes, and illicit drugs). Injection drug use may result in the development of acute and chronic wounds. The person who uses illicit drugs can have multiple health problems that may have an impact on wound healing. This issue summarizes care for the obese individual and the person who has a history of injection drug use.

The nursing shortage and the numbers of persons who lack or have insufficient health insurance affect wound care. The nursing shortage is occurring at a time when nurses are expected to make more clinical judgments about patient care and to attain high patient care quality. Nurses in all environments of care are critical for wound care. Research has shown the benefit of registered nurses in decreasing the length of hospitalization and positively affecting quality of care [2]. In addition to changing a dressing, nurses are needed to assess wounds, determine and evaluate the plan of care, and provide patient and family teaching. Nurses must have knowledge of health insurance in terms of wound care coverage. Persons who lack or have insufficient health insurance usually do not have primary care and have greater unmet health needs, an increased risk of decline in overall health, and higher rates of hospitalization. States struggle with the numbers of persons to place in Medicaid-type programs, the services that are allowed on these plans, and how to balance their budgets. Cuts in programs affect wound care services in all settings.

Quality wound care requires matching the appropriate dressing to the wound. New products cycle onto the market, and former products remain or are removed. Staying familiar with wound care products can be challenging. Wound care decisions should not be random but based on evidence of attributes of the dressing. Wounds that are necrotic generally need debridement. Debridement decreases the bacteria in the wound and facilitates healing. To relieve pressure on a wound, bed support surfaces may need to be considered. The patient must always remain active in wound care decisions. The ideal product is not ideal if the family cannot afford it or is uncomfortable in handling it. Waste must be decreased. Patient safety is a cornerstone in care planning. This issue presents updates about wound care products, bed support surfaces, and debridement.

No matter what the wound type or treatment, the patient and family are central to all care decisions. Wounds are associated with pain, changes in life style, odor, embarrassment, altered body image, and decreased employment and social activities. Literacy level of the patient will determine how information is taught. Reading ability is on average three to five grade levels below the number of grades of school completed [3]. The reading level of patient teaching materials and the best way to do patient teaching must be considered. Information and decisions about wound care must flow among the patient, family, nurses, and other care providers. Cooperation among clinicians is critical. Health promotion must be stressed. Resources must be used efficiently. Nurses need to focus on the entire episode of care and anticipate predictable patterns in the course of wound care.

In summary, this wound care issue provides information about wound physiology and microbiology, types of wounds, conditions associated with wounds, and wound care treatment. Knowledge about wounds and their treatment will continue to evolve. Although the challenge to provide quality evidenced-based care is ever present, nurses in cooperation with other health care professionals positively affect wound care for persons with multiple physical and psychosocial health problems.

Barbara Pieper, PhD, RN, CS, CWOCN, FAAN
Professor, College of Nursing
Wayne State University
5557 Cass Avenue
Detroit, MI 48202, USA
and
Nurse Practitioner, Detroit Receiving Hospital
4201 St. Antoine Blvd.
Detroit, MI 48201, USA

E-mail address: bpieper@wayne.edu

References

[1] Huckstadt AA. The experience of hospitalized elderly patients. J Gerontol Nurs 2002;28:25–9.
[2] Needleman J, Buerhaus P, Mattke S, et al. Nurse-staffing levels and the quality of care in hospitals. N Engl J Med 2002;346:1715–22.
[3] Lee PP. Why literacy matters. Arch Ophthalmol 1999;117:100–3.

ELSEVIER
SAUNDERS

Nurs Clin N Am 40 (2005) 191–205

NURSING
CLINICS
OF NORTH AMERICA

Overview: Acute and Chronic Wounds

JoAnne D. Whitney, PhD, RN, CWCN, FAAN

Biobehavioral Nursing and Health Systems, University of Washington,
School of Nursing, Box 357266, University of Washington, School of Nursing,
Seattle, WA 98195, USA

Tissue injury is an inevitability of life. From the time we are young and sustain frequent cuts and scrapes to later years when surgery, trauma, or illness may result in more extensive tissue damage, we repeatedly experience the cycle of tissue damage–tissue repair. In most cases, wounds heal after an unimpeded and largely uneventful course. However, the healing process is not perfect, and healing impairments do occur. For individuals with wounds that persist and do not follow a normal healing trajectory, there are serious health concerns and quality of life issues. The magnitude and incidence of nonhealing or slow healing wounds are increasing as the population ages and chronic health conditions associated with wounds such as venous hypertension and diabetes become more prevalent. The most common types of chronic wounds are classified as venous, pressure, or neuropathic ulcers, which together account for 70% of all chronic wounds [1]. Statistics on chronic wound prevalence vary, however reports indicate that 0.2% to 1% of the population in developed countries suffer from venous ulcers, 0.5% from pressure ulcers, and 5% to 10% of people with diabetes experience neuropathic ulcers [2–4]. Presently, wounds are categorized broadly as acute or chronic, with specific wound types in each major category. At the advent of injury, all wounds can be considered acute regardless of cause. Accidents, trauma, burns, and surgery are events that precipitate acute wounds. Wound closure and the establishment of a functional result within an acceptable amount of time characterize acute wounds [5]. The healing process or trajectory can be depicted graphically as the percentage of the wound healed over time [6]. According to the present definition, wounds are considered chronic when healing time does not follow the expected course or fall within the range of what is considered a normal healing trajectory. The entire process is prolonged, and wounds diagnosed or categorized as chronic

---

E-mail address: joiewhit@u.washington.edu

doi:10.1016/j.cnur.2004.09.002   *nursing.theclinics.com*

often resist attempts at treatment. In addition, the quality of tissue may be poor, and a functional closure is not achieved so the wounds may reoccur. In terms of the healing trajectory, the curve is shifted away from normal, indicating the delay in healing that typifies chronic wounds [1].

The basic physiologic responses to acute injury have been understood for some time. More detailed knowledge of cellular and intracellular responses to injury has recently developed. Understanding of the biologic intricacies of repair particularly at the molecular level continues to advance and inform the development of wound therapies and management strategies. It is through this growing description and knowledge of normal tissue repair that differences in the biology of nonhealing wounds has become clearer. These differences help explain variations in the healing trajectory of nonhealing wounds and offer promise for future treatments.

The process of tissue repair

The process of wound healing after full thickness injury is characterized by cell and tissue responses that can be grouped into major phases that include (1) hemostasis, inflammatory and proliferative cellular responses, and (2) synthesis of extracellular matrix consisting of new blood vessels, collagen, connective and epithelial tissue, and subsequent remodeling of this newly formed tissue. There are differences in the extent of repair depending on the type of tissue that is damaged and the depth of injury. Superficial or partial thickness injuries primarily require regeneration of new epithelium and minimal connective tissue synthesis, whereas full thickness, open wounds require the synthesis of new vessels, collagen, epithelium, and contractile forces to achieve closure.

Hemostasis, inflammatory and proliferative responses

Reestablishment of hemostasis is the physiologic goal of the body and the first major response to tissue injury. Hemostasis is achieved through the activation of the clotting cascade that is initiated when platelets are exposed to collagen from damaged blood vessels. Vasoconstriction and platelet aggregation follow, and the deposition of the fibrin clot establishes a provisional extracellular matrix [7]. The provisional matrix provides a scaffold for cell migration and entry into the injured area.

The inflammatory and proliferative cellular responses begin 24 to 48 hours after injury with the infiltration of neutrophils and then macrophages (peaking at approximately 5 days), fibroblasts (peaking at 7–9 days), and lymphocytes (peaking at approximately day 7) into the area of injury. Growth factors combined with adhesion molecules play critical roles in orchestrating and enabling the cellular responses required for successful healing. A large number of growth factors have been identified and linked to healing. Throughout the healing process, growth factors are released by cells central to the repair process. Initially, the injury response causes platelets to release growth factors and neutrophils and macrophages to migrate to the injury site, which stimulates and regulates the proliferation, migration, and local function of the cells that are critical to healing [8]. Platelets release platelet-derived growth factor (PDGF), transforming growth factors (TGF)-α and -β, fibroblast growth factor (FGF)-2, and epidermal and endothelial growth factors; fibroblasts produce vascular endothelial growth factor (VEGF) and fibroblast growth factor (FGF) [9]. Macrophages, cells required for healing, secrete TGF-α and -β, PDGF, interleukin (IL)-1, and basic FGF [10]. Lymphocytes modulate healing through the release of several growth factors including IL-1 through 10, tumor necrosis factor (TNF), fibroblast-activating factor, and macrophage-activating and in-hibitory factors. These and other growth factors regulate several aspects of fibroblast, endothelial, and keratinocyte growth and function, including stimulation of cell migration, proliferation, and synthesis of the new tissue.

Cells migrate to the area of injury under the influence of growth factors. The migratory process is assisted by the expression of cellular adhesion molecules on the surface of recruited cells and on other cells, for example endothelial cells that line capillaries. Cell adhesion molecules and receptors interact with growth factors and other proteins in the extracellular environment, resulting in the transmission of information that signals cell differentiation, growth, and a number of additional cell functions [11]. Integrins are cellular adhesion molecules that are highly involved in the healing process. They participate in platelet aggregation, cell migration and immune activity, matrix deposition, and wound contraction [12]. Cellular migration is also facilitated by matrix metalloproteinases or MMP, zinc-dependent enzymes that are present during normal healing. Twenty-three MMP enzymes have been identified in humans and are divided into six subgroups (collagenases, gelatinases, stomelysins, matrilysins, membrane type, and other) based on their structure and the substrate on which they act [13]. They are produced in response to injury by neutrophils, macrophages, fibroblasts, endothelial cells, and keratinocytes and are not generally present in normal resting tissue [14]. The MMP enzymes assist fibroblasts, endothelial cells, and keratinocytes to migrate within the wound by breaking down debris and by specific cleavage of extracellular matrix proteins as the tissue repairs and remodels [15]. MMP enzymes are kept in balance by specific inhibitors that bind to the MMP, called tissue inhibitors of metalloproteinases (TIMPs) [13]. The TIMP effectively create an antiprotease shield that prevents over-production of MMP during normal healing.

Synthesis of new tissues and remodeling

New tissues that are synthesized during repair include capillaries and connective tissue, consisting largely of collagen and epithelium. The sequencing of these newly forming tissues is overlapping, and their synthesis is interdependent. For example, new vessels are required to support the forming matrix, which in turn supports the newly established capillary network [16]. New capillary growth closely follows the entry of fibroblasts into the wound and results from endothelial budding of existing capillaries in tissues that surround the wound. There are a number of factors that stimulate angiogenesis, including growth factors released by macrophages and keratinocytes, the hypoxic, high-lactate wound environment, and low concentrations of reactive oxygen species that are produced normally during repair [17,18]. New capillaries are established as endothelial cells grow and extend toward hypoxic zones in wounds. The endothelial cells develop into capillary buds and join with other similar buds forming new capillary loops and re-establishing blood flow [19].

Epithelium begins to regenerate early after injury, and an epithelial seal of a closed surgical wound is present within 24 to 48 hours. The new epithelium completes closure, providing protection to the new collagen matrix and acting as a barrier to environmental insults and bacterial invasion. The migration of epithelial cells across a wound provides protection against the entry of bacteria into the wound and loss of fluid. Within 24 to 48 hours of wounding, epithelial marginal basal cells enlarge, flatten, undergo mitosis, and migrate over the defect [20,21]. When the layer is complete, the cells again divide, forming another layer of epithelium. Hair follicles also serve as a source of epithelial cells, forming islands of epithelial tissue in wounds. The cells migrate a distance of 1 cell diameter per hour [22]. Wound desiccation and eschar on the wound surface act as deterrents to epithelial cell movement. In wounds allowed to heal in a moist, protected environment, epithelial cells migrate on top of the wound. By contrast, wounds epithelialize by cell migration under eschar that forms when a wound is allowed to become dry. Early studies by Winter [22] showed that the rate of epithelialization in surgical epidermal wounds that were kept moist was twice that of wounds exposed to air, demonstrating that moist healing is a faster and more economical process than healing in a dry wound bed.

The extracellular matrix initially consists of fibrin, fibronectin, and hyaluronic acid but is eventually replaced with collagen [8]. Collagen, the major component of tissue repair, is synthesized by fibroblasts. The collagen molecule is a triple helix consisting of three polypeptide chains, each a single, distinct gene product [23]. The repeating amino acid sequence of the triple helical domain is Xaa-Yaa-glycine, where Xaa is often proline, and Yaa is often the modified, hydroxylated amino acid 4-hydroxyproline. There are at least 20 distinct genetic types of collagen encoded from one or more of 30 genes, in which I, II, and III are the major types involved in cutaneous healing [24]. Type II is exclusive to cartilaginous tissues; types I and III are found in dermal tissue; and type I is the most abundant, accounting for 80% of dermal dry weight. The intracellular process of collagen biosynthesis begins with selective transcription of the specific collagen gene. For type I collagen, the mRNA encoding the pre-pro-α collagen polypeptides is translated on the ribosomes into α chains. Posttranslational modification of some of the amino acid residues occurs in the endoplasmic reticulum; proline and lysine residues are converted to hydroxyproline and hydrox-ylysine through enzymatic attachment of an oxygen atom by the hydroxylases. Activity of the enzyme involved in the hydroxylation requires the presence of several cofactors: ferrous ions, 2-oxoglutarate, molecular oxygen, and ascorbate. A local tissue oxygen tension of 25 mm Hg is needed to support this reaction at half its maximal rate [25]. The modified single procollagen α chains then assemble into a triple helix, the tropocollagen molecule that is secreted into the extracellular space. Once outside of the cell, the tropocollagen molecules form cross-links and combine into collagen fibers.

The synthesis of collagen begins 3 to 5 days after the initial injury, and it continues to be produced and remodeled over several weeks and months as it orients along lines of tension and is reconfigured into a stronger tighter matrix [26]. After injury, collagen ultimately provides strength and support to tissues through its deposition and cross-linking.

Wound contraction occurs in wounds closing by secondary intention. It is the active process by which the area of a full thickness wound is decreased by the movement of the whole thickness of surrounding skin [15]. During this process new tissue is not formed; rather, the wound area is reduced and covered by the inward movement of existing tissue at the wound edge. The mechanism by which contraction occurs continues to be explored. Myofibroblasts, cells with microfibril and microtubule components, present in large numbers within the granulation tissue were thought to be the primary cells responsible for contraction [27]. In animal models [22,28], myofibroblasts were identified in granulating skin wounds and shown to respond similarly to smooth muscle in response to pharmacologic stimulants and relaxants. Further research [29] suggested that contraction results from the combined effects of vascular supply, fibroblasts, and the connective tissue matrix within the healing wound. More recently, a study [30] using an animal model determined that myofibroblasts are not required for wounds to contract. Subsequently, a study of contracting pilonidal wounds in humans by Berry et al [31] indicated also that myofibroblasts are not responsible. Instead, the study indicated that fibroblasts are the important cells and influence contraction by reorganizing collagen fibrils into thick collagen fibers that compact and pull on surrounding tissues.

Changes in the healing trajectory and microenvironment in chronic wounds

The complexity of processes that occur to produce normal healing and alterations to these processes that occur in impaired healing cannot be overstated. Healing is affected by many factors and can be viewed from several perspectives, which span the entire person and his or her environment to the cellular level and the local wound environment. From the perspective of the whole person there are several factors that increase vulnerability to impaired healing. Many factors are associated with specific diagnoses, for example, diabetes-related neuroendocrine or venous hypertension pathology, changes in health status such as protein-energy malnutrition, or medication-related immune function suppression. A detailed discussion of the multiple systemic influences on healing is beyond the scope of this review, and readers are referred to recent, informative papers [32,33].

At the level of the wound microenvironment, it has become apparent that chronic wounds can be differentiated from acute wounds on the basis of variations in the normal wound biology that manifest as changes in the local wound profile of important mediators of repair and related cellular responses. Specific areas targeted and identified in studies have increased our understanding of biologic changes that lead to delayed or failed wound healing. Major gains in knowledge have been made in identifying acute and chronic wound differences in terms of bacterial, growth factor, and protease profiles, and inflammatory responses. In chronic wounds these responses are inter-related and often interdependent.

Bacteria in chronic wounds

Chronic wounds are colonized with large numbers of microorganisms that play a role in prolonging inflammation and delaying healing [34]. It has been appreciated for some time that a lack of bacterial equilibrium is associated with delayed healing and wound chronicity, although the mechanisms linking the two are not well understood [35]. Conceptually and quantitatively, bacterial balance is a state of equilibrium defined by a bacterial level below 10^5 organisms/g of tissue [36]. Because of its virulence, β-hemolytic *Streptococcus* is the one organism that is problematic at levels below 10^5 organisms/g of tissue [37]. Early research [34,38,39] demonstrated that bacteria levels exceeding 10^5 are associated with poor healing in both surgical and chronic wounds. Open wounds and exposed granulation tissue offer an opportunity for bacterial entry and proliferation. Even though clinical signs of infection may not be evident, high wound bacterial loads are likely to prevent healing [40]. Once these bacteria have become well established in the wound, restoration of a healthy granulation bed is needed to achieve closure. This has prompted recognition of the importance of wound bed preparation as a method to create a bacterially balanced, healthy wound base before using treatments that are often costly and potentially doomed to fail in a wound that is heavily colonized. This concept was implemented within the context of a trial testing growth factor treatment of pressure ulcers (N = 61 patients) [41]. All ulcers were brought into bacterial balance before beginning the growth factor therapy with sharp debridement. Ninety-six percent of the ulcers remained in bacterial balance during the 5 weeks of the trial, with levels lower than 10^2 bacteria/g of tissue. Browne et al [40] illustrated the importance of decreasing the bacterial burden in wounds in a small trial (N = 8) using a skin substitute to treat neuropathic ulcers. Despite the absence of clinical signs of infection, 5 of the 8 ulcers had bacterial loads confirmed by biopsy that were equal to or greater than 10^5. Furthermore, decreased healing rates were associated with higher bacterial levels.

There is growing understanding and documentation of the variety of microflora that exist in chronic ulcers. Organisms commonly found in venous ulcers include staphylococci, streptococci, enterococci, the gram-negative bacilli *Pseudomonas* sp, *Enterobacter cloacae*, and *Escherichia coli*, and the anerobe *Peptococcus magnus* [42,43]. *P. aeruginosa, Providencia*, peptococci, *Bacteroides* sp, and *Clostridium* sp are reported present in nonhealing pressure ulcers [3]. In neuropathic ulcers, *Staphylococcus aureus* and *E. coli* were reported as the bacteria most commonly isolated [44]. Anaerobic bacteria have also been reported in the deeper tissues of venous ulcers, and their presence is associated with inhibition of fibroblasts and keratinocytes [45]. This provides some evidence that suggests a mechanism of bacterial impairment of the cells that are needed in healing. Recently, using polymerase chain reaction molecular analysis, a case study [46] demonstrated a more complete picture of organisms present in a venous ulcer of a patient without clinical signs of infection. Swab and tissue biopsies isolated four organisms, whereas molecular analysis identified five additional bacterial species. The clinical significance of these findings is not clear, but it seems an important step toward using new technologies that will provide more comprehensive characterization of the bacterial profile in chronic wounds and potentially help define more specific and effective treatments.

Growth factor and inflammatory changes in chronic wounds

Compared with acute wounds, nonhealing wounds show differences in the presence and quantity of growth factors as well as cellular responses to growth factors. In some cases the growth factor is present but wound cells lack receptors capable of responding to the growth factor; in other cases the type of growth factor and its amount in the wound is altered [47,48]. In either case, orchestration of the healing process is changed and deviates from a normal course.

Differences in growth factor presence (increased or decreased levels) and activity have been reported in most types of chronic wounds, including venous ulcers, neuropathic ulcers, and pressure ulcers [49]. One notable difference is the presence of higher levels of growth factors that promote inflammation. Increases in inflammatory growth factors such as TNF-α,

IL-1α, and IL-6 have been reported in venous ulcers [50,51]. In nonhealing areas of burns, increases in TNF-α, IL-6, and IL-8 are also documented [52]. Prolonged inflammation is associated with increased production of reactive oxygen species by neutrophils and increased expression of proteases (further detailed below) that promote a cycle of tissue destruction rather than synthesis [1]. It has also been observed that the presence of proinflammatory growth factors declined when venous ulcers began to heal, indicating removal of inhibitory influences on healing [50]. Decreases in growth factors involved in recruitment and stimulation of cells needed for repair (PDGF, TGF-β1, IGF-1, and FGF) have also been documented [53–56].

Recent interest in studying aspects of angiogenesis and the presence of VEGF in chronic wounds was prompted in part by the recognition of the critical role of VEGF in stimulating new capillary growth and issues of ischemia in chronic wounds [57]. Work by Drinkwater et al [58] to determine VEGF levels in ulcers showed that its concentration in wound fluid was significantly higher in venous ulcers that were nonhealing compared with those healing satisfactorily. There was no difference in the concentration of VEGF receptors (VEGF-R1) between nonhealing and healing ulcers. Lower levels of VEGF had been expected; higher levels suggest an increase in stimulus for new vessel growth without a significant response. High levels of VEGF have also been reported in the plasma of patients with venous ulcers [59]. A similar situation was observed in chronic pressure ulcers. Biopsies of the necrotic central area, granulation tissue, and the surrounding skin of these ulcers showed moderate VEGF levels in skin and the necrotic area and high levels in granulation tissue [60]. This supports the idea that the observed lack of angiogenesis is not caused by VEGF deficiency but by some other factor. It is also illustrates the complex nature and variation in pathology involved in nonhealing wounds.

How growth factors become unbalanced in chronic wounds is not yet completely clear. Current ideas include the concept of growth factor trapping in tissues, where it is proposed that growth factors become bound to protein macromolecules or are prevented from locating to the wound by fibrin deposits or cuffs, as in the case of venous ulcers [8,61]. Another possible mechanism associated with decreased growth factor levels is an increase in proteases that in turn degrade growth factors [1].

It is also likely that not only growth factor imbalances but a lack of ability of cells to respond to growth factor signals is a factor in delayed healing. Senescence is the process or condition of growing old, and chronic wounds have increased numbers of senescent cells that have lessened or lost the capability to respond to growth factors [47]. Senescent cells may also be in a state of cell cycle arrest (unresponsive to signaling proteins), a new concept that may help to explain healing failure or the lack of treatment response observed in chronic wounds [62]. Deficient cellular response is illustrated by the decreased proliferative responses of fibroblasts to stimulation by TGF-β1, taken from patients with advanced stage venous ulcers [63]. These cells are shown to have reduced expression of receptors and abnormalities in intracellular signaling pathways [64,65]. A similar lack of responsiveness and senescence is reported in cells obtained from certain locations within pressure ulcers [66]. On the other hand, other studies [67] report findings in which venous ulcer fibroblasts did not show signs of senescence in terms of the cells' ability to replicate or attach to the extracellular matrix. Hence, the exact nature, extent, and impact of senescence in chronic wounds require continued study to provide a more complete picture. Recent research [68] indicates that it may be possible to identify whether wounds have high numbers of senescent or arrested cells by detecting levels of cyclin-dependent kinases and cyclin proteins that direct cells through the cell cycle. This level of wound analysis could be very useful in the design of future treatments and related studies in which therapies target and rely on specific cell responses to accomplish healing.

Proteolytic changes in chronic wounds

Similar to growth factors, imbalances in MMP and other protein-degrading enzymes are documented in wounds with delayed healing compared with normally healing wounds. In the presence of elevated proteolytic enzymes or MMP that are not kept in normal balance through TIMP activity, the balance is shifted toward increased proteolysis. As currently understood, the increased levels of these enzymes are likely responsible for the degradation of growth factors and extracellular matrix proteins that characterize chronic wounds [69].

Compared with acutely healing wounds, 30-fold increases in proteases have been reported in wound fluid sampled from chronic wound subtypes including venous, arterial, neuropathic, and pressure-related ulcers [70]. In pressure ulcers, increased amounts of MMP-8 (collagenase-2) have been measured [71]. Wound fluid from venous ulcers is reported to have increased MMP-2 (gelatinase-A) and MMP-9 (gelatinase-B) levels [72,73]. Results from biopsies taken from the edge, base, and surrounding intact skin of chronic venous ulcers documented that MMP-9 was present in the cells located in the ulcer bed but not the wound periphery [74]. This finding differed from the normally healing comparison of wounds in which MMP-9 was present in the advancing epithelium. The findings suggest that increased or decreased distribution of protease-producing cells in specific wound areas may be also be a factor that impairs healing in chronic wounds.

In patients with diabetes, a number of alterations from normal appear to operate. MMP-2 levels in wound fluid from patients with diabetes-related wounds were significantly higher than those measured in acute wounds [75]. Furthermore, fibroblasts taken from nonwounded skin areas in patients with diabetes show elevated production of MMP-2 and MMP-3 (strome-lysin-1), suggesting underlying pathology in resident fibroblasts even without tissue injury [76]. Protease disregulation has also been demonstrated in tissue biopsies from chronic diabetes-related wounds. In tissue taken from the center of neuropathic ulcers, levels of MMP-1, MMP-2, MMP-8, and MMP-9 were all found to be significantly increased above those found in traumatic wounds [77]. Additionally, the study documented reduced expression of TIMP-2 compared with levels from the traumatic wounds, demonstrating the imbalances that impede repair. Other factors are also present in diabetes that potentially reduce the ability to heal, including (1) neutral endopeptidase, an MMP involved in neuroinflammatory signaling and epithelial repair that is elevated in neuropathic ulcers [78,79], and (2) higher amounts of insulin-degrading enzyme in neuropathic ulcers, which degrades insulin as well as growth factors [80]. Again, the emerging evidence illustrates the complexity of impaired healing and the combined influence of several pathologic factors in limiting repair.

The increased proteolytic profile of chronic wounds can be explained in part by increased numbers of neutrophils [69]. Neutrophils produce and store a number of enzymes used to control or clear bacteria and debris in injured tissues, including collagenase, which degrades collagen, and elastase, which is able to degrade growth factors PDGF and TGF-β [81]. The consequences of the prolonged presence of these phagocytic cells are ongoing wound inflammation and lack of matrix synthesis. Recent research [82] comparing normal tissue samples with those taken from granulating areas of pressure ulcers demonstrated the presence of extensive numbers of neutrophils and irregularities in the wound matrix in the pressure ulcers. The presence of large numbers of neutrophils is consistent with the increased proteases within chronic wounds and the overall concept of tissue breakdown in excess of synthesis.

Implications for managing chronic wounds

No single approach or therapy has successfully solved the dilemma of treating intractable, slowly healing, or nonhealing wounds. However, our improved awareness of factors differentiating chronic wounds from those that heal normally helps to account for the lack of uniform success in wound treatments. Greater understanding of the physiologic alterations present in chronic wounds has helped to develop and reconsider specific management strategies. Bacterial imbalances, increased presence of inflammatory cells and proinflammatory growth factors, increased protease synthesis and release by wound cells, reductions in TIMP, and cells that are incapable of responding to interventions are implicated in the multifaceted picture of chronic wounds. Better understanding of these chronic wound features and the relationships among factors that must be considered when novel therapies are used will help to increase treatment efficacy.

Bringing the wound into a state of improved physiologic balance is critical for the successful management of chronic wounds. This is reflected in the growing emphasis on wound bed preparation that is recommended before the application of available treatments [83–85]. The concept of wound bed preparation includes the main components: debridement and removal of necrotic tissue, control of edema and exudate, and bacterial and moisture balance [35,86]. Additionally, it is critical that causes of tissue damage be evaluated and corrected as well as ensuring adequate tissue perfusion and oxygen supply [87]. By preparing the wound bed, it is possible to alter and bring into balance a number of negative influences that exist in chronic wounds, including bacteria and other sources of inflammation, proteases, and senescent cells. Detailed information on the technical aspects of wound bed preparation is available in a number of sources [35,83–86]. When wound tissue is brought toward physiologic balance, additional local and systemic treatments are likely to have a greater chance of supporting healing and subsequent successful wound closure.

Future therapies are likely to be directed at manipulating the local environment and cellular responses in chronic wounds [88]. Work will continue to evaluate the efficacy of a number of growth factors, the most effective combinations or sequencing of growth factors, methods to control excessive inflammatory cell functions and inhibit proteolytic forces, the application of gene therapy to wounds, development of skin equivalents, and the efficacy of adjunctive therapies [48,87,89,90]. Topical use of nerve growth factor to treat pressure ulcers is an example of an area of current interest and study [88,91]. In addition to these efforts, translation of knowledge and optimum delivery of chronic wound care are essential. There is increased recognition for the necessity of management protocols that are informed by the growing scientific base for treatment, evidence-based guidelines and standards that reflect current best practices [92]. In addition, interdisciplinary teams and networks of wound care centers are regarded as vital to the coordination of care and ability to document and evaluate patient outcomes [47,93]. Although there is much to be done to improve outcomes in patients who suffer from chronic wounds, the future looks promising. The efforts of basic and clinical scientists in combination with expert interdisciplinary teams armed with new knowledge offers great potential for reducing the burden of chronic wounds.

References

[1] Nwomeh BC, Yager DR, Cohen IK. Physiology of the chronic wound. Clin Plast Surg 1998; 25:341–56.

[2] Simka M, Majewski E. The social and economic burden of venous leg ulcers: focus on the role of micronized purified flavonoid fraction adjuvant therapy. Am J Clin Dermatol 2003;4: 573–81.

[3] Thomas DR. Issues and dilemmas in the prevention and treatment of pressure ulcers: a review. J Gerontol 2001;56A:M328–40.

[4] Reiber GE. Epidemiology of foot ulcerations and amputations in diabetes. 6th edition. St Louis: Mosby; 2001.

[5] Lazarus GS, Cooper DM, Knighton DR, et al. Definitions and guidelines for assessment of wounds and evaluation of healing. Arch Dermatol 1994;130:489–93.

[6] Steed DL. Wound healing trajectories. Surg Clin North Am 2003;83(3):547–55.

[7] Clark RA. Fibrin and wound healing. Ann N Y Acad Sci 2001;936:355–67.

[8] Singer AJ, Clark RAF. Cutaneous wound healing. N Engl J Med 1999;341:738–46.

[9] Cross KJ, Mustoe TA. Growth factors in wound healing. Surg Clin North Am 2003;83: 531–45.

[10] Hopkinson I. The extracellular matrix in wound healing: collagen in wound healing. Wounds 1992;4:124–32.

[11] Frenette PS, Wagner DD. Molecular medicine: adhesion molecules–part 1. N Engl J Med 1996;334:1526–9.

[12] Mutsaers SE, Bishop JE, McGrouther G, et al. Mechanisms of tissue repair: from wound healing to fibrosis. Int J Biochem Cell Biol 1997;29:5–17.

[13] Visse R, Nagase H. Matrix metalloproteinases and tissue inhibitors of metalloproteinases. Structure, function and biochemistry. Circ Res 2003;92:827–39.

[14] Parks WC. Matrix metalloproteinases in repair. Wound Repair Regen 1999;7:423–32.

[15] Stamenkovic I. Extracellular matrix remodeling: the role of matrix metalloproteinases. J Pathol 2003;200:448–64.

[16] Hunt TK. The physiology of wound healing. Ann Emerg Med 1988;17:1265–73.

[17] Hunt TK, Hopf HW, Hussain Z. Physiology of wound healing. Adv Skin Wound Care 2000; 13(Suppl 2):S6–11.

[18] Sen CK. The general case for redox control of wound repair. Wound Repair Regen 2003;11: 431–8.

[19] Hunt TK, Goodson WH. Wound healing. In: Way LW, editor. Current surgical diagnosis and treatment. Norwalk (CT): Appleton and Lange; 1988. p. 86–97.

[20] Winter GD. Some factors affecting skin and wound healing. In: Kenedi RM, Cowden JM, editors. Bedsore biomechanics. Baltimore: University Park Press; 1976. p. 47–54.

[21] Peacock EE. Wound Repair. 3rd edition. Philadelphia: WB Saunders; 1984.

[22] Winter GD. Formation of the scab and the rate of epithelization of superficial wounds in the skin of the young domestic pig. Nature 1962;193:293–4.

[23] Miller EJ, Gay S. Collagen structure and function. In: Cohen IK, Dieglemann RF, Lindblad WJ, editors. Wound healing biochemical and clinical aspects. Philadelphia: WB Saunders; 1992. p. 130–51.

[24] Diegelmann RF. Collagen metabolism. Wounds 2001;13:177–82.

[25] Hunt TK. Basic principles of wound healing. J Trauma 1990;30(Suppl 12):S122–8.

[26] Enquist IF, Adamson RJ. Collgen synthesis and lysis in healing wounds. Minn Med 1965;48: 1695–8.

[27] Majno G, Gabbiani G, Hirshcel BJ, et al. Contraction of granulation tissue in vitro: similarity to smooth muscle. Science 1971;173:548–50.

[28] Rudolph R, Woodward M, Hurn I. Ultrastructure of active versus passive contracture of wounds. Surg Gynecol Obstet 1980;151:396–400.

[29] Ehrlich HP. The role of connective tissue matrix in hypertrophic scar contracture. In: Hunt TK, Heppenstall RB, Pines E, Rovee D, editors. Soft and hard tissue repair. New York: Prager; 1984. p. 533–53.

[30] Ehrlich HP, Keefer KA, Myers RL, et al. Vanadate and the absence of myofibroblasts in wound contraction. Arch Surg 1999;134:494–501.

[31] Berry DP, Harding KG, Stanton MR, et al. Human wound contraction: collagen organization, fibroblasts, and myofibroblasts. Plast Reconstr Surg 1998;102:124–31.

[32] Greenhalgh DG. Wound healing and diabetes mellitus. Clin Plast Surg 2003;30:37–45.

[33] Burns JL, Mancoll JS, Phillips LG. Impairments to wound healing. Clin Plast Surg 2003;30: 47–56.

[34] Bowler PG. Wound pathophysiology, infection and therapeutic options. Ann Med 2002;34: 419–27.

[35] Falanga V. The chronic wound: impaired healing and solutions in the context of wound bed preparation. Blood Cells Mol Dis 2004;32:88–94.

[36] Robson MC, Heggers JP. Bacterial quantification of open wounds. Mil Med 1969;134: 19–24.

[37] Robson MC, Heggers JP. The B-hemolytic streptococcus. J Surg Res 1969;9:289–92.

[38] Liedberg NCF, Reiss E, Artz CP. The effect of bacteria on the take of split thickness skin grafts in rabbits. Ann Surg 1955;142:92–7.

[39] Bendy RH, Nuccio PA, Wolfe E, et al. Relationship of quantitative wound bacterial counts to healing of decubiti: effects of gentamicin. Antimicrob Agents Chemother 1964; 4:147–55.

[40] Browne AC, Vearncombe M, Sibbald RG. High bacterial load in asymptomatic diabetic patients with neurotrophic ulcers retards wound healing after application of dermagraft. Ostomy Wound Manage 2001;47:44–9.

[41] Robson MC, Mannari RJ, Smith PD. Maintenance of wound bacterial balance. Am J Surg 1999;178:399–402.

[42] Brook I, Frazier EH. Aerobic and anaerobic microbiology of chronic venous ulcers. Int J Dermatol 1998;37:426–8.

[43] Hansson C, Hoborn J, Moller A, et al. The microbial flora in venous leg ulcers without clinical signs of infection using a validated standardized microbiological technique. Acta Derm Venereol 1995;75:24–30.

[44] McLigeyo OS, Otieno SL. Diabetic ulcers—a clinical and bacteriological study. West Afr J Med 1990;9:135–8.

[45] Stephens P, Wall IB, Wilson MJ, et al. Anaerobic cocci populating the deep tissues of chronic wounds impair cellular wound healing responses in vitro. Br J Dermatol 2003;148:456–66.

[46] Hill KE, Davies CE, Wilson MJ, et al. Molecular analysis of the microflora in chronic venous leg ulceration. J Med Microbiol 2003;52:365–9.

[47] Harding KG, Morris HL, Patel GK. Science, medicine and the future: healing chronic wounds. BMJ 2002;324:160–3.

[48] Goldman R. Growth factors and chronic wound healing: past, present, and future. Adv Skin Wound Care 2004;17:24–35.

[49] Cooper DM, Yu EZ, Hennessey P, et al. Determination of endogenous cytokines in chronic wounds. Am Surg 1994;219:688–92.

[50] Trengrove N, Langton S, Stacey M. Biochemical analysis of wound fluid from nonhealing and healing chronic leg ulcers. Wound Repair Regen 1996;4:234–9.

[51] Trengrove NJ, Bielefeldt-Ohmann H, Stacey MC. Mitogenic activity and cytokine levels in non-healing and healing chronic leg ulcers. Wound Repair Regen 2000;8:13–25.

[52] Henry G, Garner WL. Inflammatory mediators in wound healing. Surg Clin North Am 2003;83:483–507.

[53] Pierce GF, Tarpley JE, Tseng J, et al. Detection of platelet-derived growth factor (PDGF)-AA in actively healing human wounds treated with recombinant PDGF-BB and absence of PDGF in chronic nonhealing wounds. J Clin Invest 1995;96:1336–50.

[54] Shukla A, Dubey MP, Srivastava R, et al. Differential expression of proteins during healing of cutaneous wounds in experimental normal and chronic models. Biochem Biophys Res Commun 1998;144:434–9.

[55] Jude EB, Bulmer BJ, Coulton AJM, et al. Transforming growth factor-beta 1,2,3 and receptor type I and II in diabetic foot ulcers. Diabet Med 2002;19:440–7.

[56] Blakytny R, Jude EB, Gibson JM, et al. Lack of insulin-like growth factor 1 (IGF 1) in the basal ketatinocyte layer of diabetic skin and diabetic foot ulcers. J Pathol 2000;190: 589–94.

[57] Cross KJ, Mustoe TA. Growth factors in wound healing. Surg Clin North Am 2003;83: 531–45.

[58] Drinkwater S, Burnand KG, Ding R, et al. Increased but ineffectual angiogenic drive in nonhealing venous leg ulcers. J Vasc Surg 2003;38:1106–12.

[59] Shoab SS, Scur JH, Coleridge-Smith PD. Increased plasma vascular endothelial growth factor among patients with chronic venous disease. J Vasc Surg 1998;28:535–40.

[60] Pufe T, Paulsen F, Petersen W, et al. The angiogenic peptide vascular endothelial growth factor (VEGF) is expressed in chronic sacral pressure ulcers. J Pathol 2003;200:130–6.

[61] Falanga V, Eaglstein WH. The "trap" hypothesis of venous ulceration. Lancet 1993;341: 1006–8.

[62] Vande Berg JS, Robson MC. Arresting cell cycles and the effect on wound healing. Surg Clin North Am 2003;83:509–20.

[63] Lal BK, Saito S, Pappas PJ, et al. Altered proliferative responses of dermal fibroblasts to TGF-β1 may contribute to chronic venous stasis ulcer. J Vasc Surg 2003;37:1285–93.

[64] Kim BC, Kim HT, Park SH, et al. Fibroblasts from chronic wounds show altered TGF-β-Signaling and decreased TGF-β- Type II receptor expression. J Cell Physiol 2003;195:331–6.

[65] Cowin AJ, Holding HN, Dunaiski CA, et al. Effect of healing on the expression of transforming growth factor βs and their receptors in chronic venous leg ulcers. J Invest Dermatol 2001;117:1282–9.

[66] Van de Berg JS, Rudolph R, Hollan C, et al. Fibroblast senescence in pressure ulcers. Wound Repair Regen 1998;6:38–49.

[67] Stephens P, Cook H, Hilton J, et al. An analysis of replicative senescence in dermal fibroblasts derived from chronic leg wounds predicts that telomerase therapy would fail to reverse their disease-specific cellular and proteolytic phenotype. Exp Cell Res 2003;283: 22–35.

[68] Van de Berg JS, Rose MA, Payne WG, et al. Significance of cell cycle for wound stratification in clinical trials: analysis of a pressure ulcer clinical trial utilizing cyclin D/cdk4. Wound Repair Regen 2003;11:11–8.

[69] Yager DR, Nwomeh BC. The proteolytic environment of chronic wounds. Wound Repair Regen 1999;7:433–41.

[70] Trengrove NJ, Stacey MC, Macauley S, et al. Analysis of the acute and chronic wound environments: the role of proteases and their inhibitors. Wound Repair Regen 1999;7: 442–52.

[71] Nwomeh BC, Liang HX, Cohen IK, et al. MMP-8 is the predominant collagenase in healing wounds and nonhealing ulcers. J Surg Res 81:189–95.

[72] Wysocki AB, Staiano-Coico L, Grinnell F. Wound fluid from chronic leg ulcers contains elevated levels of metalloproteinases MMP-2 and MMP-9. J Invest Derm 1993;101:64–8.

[73] Weckroth M, Vaheri A, Lauharanta J, et al. Matrix metalloproteinases, gelatinase and collagenase, in chronic leg ulcers. J Invest Dermatol 1996;106:1119–24.

[74] Mirastschijski U, Impola U, Jahkola T, et al. Ectopic localization of matrix metalloproteinases-9 in chronic cutaneous wounds. Hum Pathol 2002;33:355–64.

[75] Wall SJ, Bevan D, Thomas DW, et al. Differential expression of matrix metalloproteinases during impaired wound healing of the diabetes mouse. J Invest Dermatol 2002;119:91–8.

[76] Wall SJ, Sampson MJ, Levell N, et al. Elevated matrix metalloproteinase-t and –3 production from human diabetic dermal fibroblasts. Br J Dermatol 2003;149:13–6.

[77] Lobman R, Ambrosch A, Schultz G, et al. Expression of matrix-metalloproteinases and their inhibitors in the wounds of diabetic and non-diabetic patients. Diabetologia 2002;45:1011–6.

[78] Antzana MA, Sullivan SR, Usui ML, et al. Neutral endopeptidase activity is increased in the skin of subjects with diabetic ulcers. J Invest Dermatol 2002;119:1400–4.

[79] Spenny ML, Muangman P, Sullivan SR, et al. Neutral endopeptidase inhibition in diabetic wound repair. Wound Repair Regen 2002;10:295–301.

[80] Duckworth WC, Fawcett J, Reddy S, et al. Insulin degrading activity in wound fluid. J Clin Endocrinol Metab 2004;89:847–51.

[81] Diegelmann RF, Evans MC. Wound healing: an overview of acute, fibrotic and delayed healing. Front Bio 2004;9:283–9.

[82] Diegelmann RF. Excessive neutrophils characterize chronic pressure ulcers. Wound Repair Regen 2003;11:490–5.

[83] Falanga V. Classifications for wound bed preparation and stimulation of chronic wounds. Wound Repair Regen 2000;8:347–52.

[84] Ayello EA, Cuddigan JE. Conquer chronic wounds with wound bed preparation. Nurs Pract 2004;29:8–25.

[85] Brem H, Balledux J, Sukkarieh T, et al. Healing of venous ulcers of long duration with a bilayered living skin substitute: results from a general surgery and dermatology department. Dermatol Surg 2001;27:915–9.

[86] Sibbald RB, Williamson D, Orsted HL. Preparing the wound bed–debridement, bacterial balance and moisture balance. Ostomy Wound Manage 2000;46:14–35.

[87] Schultz GS, Sibbald RG, Falanga V, et al. Wound bed preparation: a systematic approach to wound management. Wound Repair Regen 2003;11(Suppl 3):S1–28.

[88] Robson MC. Cytokine manipulation of the wound. Clin Plast Surg 2003;30:57–65.

[89] Thomas DR. The promise of topical growth factors in healing pressure ulcers. Ann Intern Med 2003;139:694–5.

[90] Petrie NC, Yao F, Eriksson E. Gene therapy in wound healing. Surg Clin North Am 2003;83: 597–616.

[91] Landi F, Aloe L, Russo A, et al. Topical treatment of pressure ulcers with nerve growth factor. Ann Intern Med 2003;139:635–41.

[92] Gottrup F, Holstein P, Jorgensen B, et al. A new concept of a multidisciplinary wound healing center and a national expert function of wound healing. Arch Surg 2001;136:765–72.

[93] Coerper S, Wicke C, Pfeffer F, et al. Documentation of 7051 chronic wounds using a new computerized system within a network of wound care centers. Arch Surg 2004;138:251–8.

ELSEVIER
SAUNDERS

Nurs Clin N Am 40 (2005) 207–216

NURSING
CLINICS
OF NORTH AMERICA

Microbiology of Chronic Leg and Pressure Ulcers: Clinical Significance and Implications for Treatment

John R. Ebright, MD[a,b,*]

[a]Department of Internal Medicine, Wayne State University School of Medicine,
Detroit Medical Center, Detroit, MI 48201, USA
[b]Division of Infectious Diseases, Harper University Hospital, 3990 John R–5 Hudson,
Detroit, MI 48201, USA

Chronic skin wounds are a major world health problem that result in distress and disability and pose a great challenge to the medical community. It is estimated that 1.3 to 3 million adults have a pressure ulcer and that the cost to achieve resolution in some patients can approach $40,000 [1]. Leg ulcers also are common and, like pressure ulcers, are especially common in the elderly. A Swedish study [2] reported that 4% to 5% of people over the age of 80 sought medical advice for leg ulcers. The pathogenesis of chronic ulcers is complex and multifactorial but usually does not include infection, at least not as an initial inciting event. In that regard, chronic ulcers are different from primary cutaneous infections such as cellulitis or ecthyma caused by *Staphylococcus aureus* or *Streptococcus pyogenes*, which rarely result in chronic ulcers. Rather, a wide variety of microorganisms predictably colonizes chronic wounds and less commonly causes a true secondary infection. The challenge to the health care provider is to recognize when the patient's chronic wound is not just colonized but truly infected and to understand how to obtain reliable microbiologic studies and provide effective treatment.

Microbiology

Studies [3,4] have demonstrated that clinically uninfected chronic leg and pressure ulcers are predictably colonized by bacteria. Moreover, multiple

* Division of Infectious Diseases, Harper University Hospital, 3990 John R–5 Hudson, Detroit, MI 48201.
  E-mail address: jebright@med.wayne.edu

0029-6465/05/$ - see front matter © 2005 Elsevier Inc. All rights reserved.
doi:10.1016/j.cnur.2004.09.003   *nursing.theclinics.com*

species are present in such wounds and include varying combinations of *S. aureus*, coagulase-negative *Staphylococcus* and *Enterococcus* sp, gram-negative bacilli such as *Escherichia coli* and *Pseudomonas aeruginosa*, and anaerobic bacteria.

Biopsies of clinically infected pressure ulcers, especially those with necrotic tissue, may isolate five to six species of bacteria, including aerobic and anaerobic organisms such as *Bacteroides* sp and anaerobic streptococci, and have a total bacterial density of more than 10^5 organisms/g of tissue. Both the density of organisms and presence of anaerobic bacteria may decrease as ulcer beds become free of necrotic tissue [5]. In a study [6] of 23 patients evaluated consecutively, bacteriological cultures from clinically infected pressure ulcers revealed an average of 4 isolates (3 aerobic and 1 anaerobic) per ulcer. Isolates included *Proteus mirabilis*, *E. coli*, enterococci, staphylococci, and *Pseudomonas* sp. Anaerobic isolates included *Peptostreptococcus* sp, *B. fragilis*, and *Clostridium perfringens*.

Several recent studies have demonstrated similar results in patients with chronic leg ulcers. Hansson et al [7] found more than one bacterial species in 86% of ulcers studied. The predominant flora included *S. aureus*, *Enterococcus faecalis*, *S. epidermidis*, *Pseudomonas* sp, gram-negative enteric organisms, and anaerobic bacteria. One or more obligate anaerobic species (*Peptococcus prevotii*, *Propionibacterium acnes*, and *Veillonella parvula*) was found in 50% of the ulcers. Fungi, including *Candida albicans*, *C. guilliermondii*, and *Rhodotorula rubra*, were found in 11% of the samples. Comparable results were found by Bowler and Davies [8] and by Brook and Frazier [9] in a retrospective review of patients with both clinically infected and clinically uninfected leg ulcers. The results of strict anaerobic isolation techniques and prolonged incubation times show that almost 60% of chronic venous leg ulcers harbor anaerobic bacteria such as *Fusobacterium* sp and peptostreptococci [10,11].

Of considerable interest are findings using molecular analysis of microflora in a chronic venous leg ulcer of a single patient. When conventional microbiologic methods were compared with molecular analysis using 16S ribosomal RNA sequences recovered by direct amplification from tissue biopsy, the molecular approach demonstrated significantly greater bacterial diversity than that of conventional culture. Three clones showing low similarity to all database sequences (the most similar sequences were from *B. ureolyticus*, *Lactosphaera pasteurii*, and *Acinetobacter lwoffi*) were not detected by culture and may therefore represent novel, previously uncultured species [12].

From the aforementioned studies, it is clear that both clinically infected and uninfected leg and pressure ulcers are populated with a complex, multispecies aerobic and anaerobic microflora. Although these conditions have been convincingly and repeatedly demonstrated by numerous and increasingly sophisticated studies, the clinical relevance of this information is proving to be much more difficult to elucidate.

Contamination, colonization, and infection

Before proceeding, it may be useful to define three terms used in literature dealing with chronic wounds [13]. A contaminated wound has transient, nonreplicating organisms on the surface. The organisms may be identified when a culture from the surface is obtained but are believed to be clinically irrelevant. A colonized wound has resident and replicating microorganisms within a wound but not invading or infecting the underlying tissue. A wound infection occurs when microorganisms cause injury to underlying tissue by invasion or toxin release or by secondary host immune response. Clinical evidence for infection includes increasing local pain, cellulitis adjacent to the ulcer, grossly purulent exudates, fever, bacteremias, or sepsis [14,15].

Clinical consequences of microorganisms within chronic wounds

Complications caused by or possibly caused by the presence of microorganisms within chronic wounds include (1) delay of wound healing even in the absence of clinical infection; (2) clinical infection, as evidenced by suppurative wounds, cellulitis, fever, bacteremia, sepsis or osteomyelitis; and (3) failure of surgical attempts to close wounds by grafting or using tissue flaps.

Additionally, it appears possible to many investigators that the complications mentioned above may occur depending on one or more of at least four microbiologic variables: (1) the presence of certain individual species of bacteria, such as *S. aureus* or *P. aeruginosa*, which are highly prone to produce pathological consequences; (2) the presence of a more complex community of microorganisms, including anaerobic bacteria, which together result in injury; (3) the presence of a high number of organisms within the wound, usually greater than 10^5 organisms/g of tissue; and (4) the location of the microorganisms, whether on the surface of the wound and detected by swab culture or within the tissue of the ulcer base and detected by biopsy or aspiration.

Delay in wound healing

Many investigators and health care providers have attempted to better understand the causes of impaired healing in chronic wounds to more effectively intervene and promote tissue repair. Hypothetically, the healing of chronically colonized but clinically uninfected wounds is delayed for multiple reasons, including local hypoxia, pericapillary deposition of fibrin, and persistent pressure, as well as direct or indirect effects of microorganisms within the wound [16–18]. It follows that if microorganisms contribute to impaired wound healing, local antibiotics or antiseptics may well be indicated to hasten recovery even in wounds that appear to be clinically uninfected. Such use of antimicrobial agents has been the focus of debate and investigation for the past several decades.

At least four mechanisms have been proposed by which microorganism might contribute to delayed healing: (1) specific, individual organism-mediated delayed healing; (2) complex, multiorganism community effect; (3) a high number of organisms per gram of tissue ("population density"); and (4) secondary, subclinical inflammatory host response.

Specific bacteria that are especially likely to impair wound healing include *S. aureus*, β-hemolytic streptococci, and *Pseudomonas* sp [19]. *Pseudomonas* sp are found in 20% to 30% of chronic venous ulcers and may release enzymes such as elastase and protease and other cytotoxic substances in the environment of chronic ulcers. Recent work by Schmidtchen et al [20] provides support for the possible role of *Pseudomonas* sp in delayed wound healing. The authors report that *P. aeruginosa*, expressing the major metalloproteinase elastase, induces degradation of complement C3, various antiproteinases, kininogens, fibroblast proteins, and proteoglycans in vitro. In addition, in ex vivo experiments using human wound fluid, skin biopsies, and plasma, elastase-producing *P. aeruginosa* isolates were shown to significantly degrade human wound fluid as well as human skin proteins. Nevertheless, the authors were unable to demonstrate a correlation between clinical severity (ulcer size and duration) and protease expression [20,21].

Multiple investigators have focused on the presence of a diverse microbial flora, including anaerobic bacteria, within wounds as an important cause of delayed wound healing. Some support for this concept was provided in a recent clinical study [19] of chronic leg ulcers. Fifty-two patients who were followed regularly in a leg ulcer clinic underwent weekly inspection and culturing using swabs after the dressings were removed. Not surprisingly, isolates included *S. aureus* (66%), β-hemolytic streptococci (22%), *Pseudomonas* sp (26%), anaerobes (16%), and mixed coliforms. The authors were not able to show a relationship between any one specific bacterial group and wound healing rate, but they found that the presence of four or more bacterial groups was associated with delayed healing.

Closely related to the importance of the number of different species of colonizing bacteria, or "bacterial community," is the postulate that the total number of organisms per gram of tissue is an important cause of delayed wound healing. Some investigators use the terms "bio-burden" or "population density" to refer to this concept. The concept of population density, which is related to the likelihood of a pathologic disease or invasive infection, dates at least to the 1950s and was recently reviewed by one of the proponents of this theory [22]. In 1956, Elek [23] injected staphylococci into normal skin and demonstrated that a mean inoculation of 7.5×10^6 organisms was necessary to produce a pustule. This was decreased by four logs if a silk suture was inserted at the site of inoculation. In 1957, Kass [24] demonstrated that 95% of patients with pyelonephritis had greater than 10^5 colony-forming units (CFUs)/mL of urine. Studies published in the mid-

1960s by the US Army Surgical Research Unit provided further support that burn wound infections correlated with colony counts of greater than 10^5 CFU/g of tissue [25,26]. A frequently quoted paper by Bendy et al [27] provided evidence that decubitus ulcers would not heal until colonizing bacteria were reduced to less than 10^6 CFU/mL. Although in all of the aforementioned studies (except possibly that of Bendy et al, in which the presence or absence of infected wounds is not clarified), population density was related to presence or absence of invasive infection; a few more recent investigators have proposed that high bacterial levels may also interfere with normal wound healing [28]. At this time, the hypothesis that bacterial density greater than 10^5 CFUs/g of clinically uninfected tissue delays wound healing is conjecture and requires further study [29].

Some investigators assert that a subclinical host response to micro-organisms colonizing the wound may interfere with recovery and slow tissue repair. The postulated injurious host response may be the relative absence of normal growth factors (platelet-derived growth factor, basic fibroblast growth factor, and epidermal growth factor) or an excess of inflammatory cytokines such as interleukin-1 and tumor necrosis factor-α. Recently, evidence has been published in support of excessive inflammatory cytokines contributing to delayed wound healing of chronic ulcers [30].

Clinical infection

Whereas all chronic wounds are colonized with bacteria, most wounds, if managed properly, will remain uninfected. Nevertheless, unfortunately, infections are well known to occur, especially with stage 3 and 4 pressure ulcers.

Most commonly, the ulcer bed and adjacent tissue are invaded, with cellulitis developing as a result. This complication is evidenced by one or more of the following: increasing local pain, edema, erythema, heat, discoloring of granulation tissue (changing from a normal "beefy" red to pale or dusky), increasing purulent discharge, and foul odor [13,15]. Less frequently, life-threatening bacteremia or sepsis may ensue [31,32]. As discussed previously, multiple types of bacteria causing clinical soft-tissue infection associated with chronic wounds frequently include S. aureus (increasingly methicillin resistant [33]), S. pyogenes [34], enterococci, gram-negative enteric organisms, Pseudomonas sp, and anaerobes such as Peptostreptococcus and Bacteroides sp [6]. In at least one study [6], the predominant bacteremic isolates were B. fragilis, Peptostreptococcus sp, P. mirabilis, and S. aureus. In 41% of the cases, bacteremia was polymicrobial.

In a 5-year prospective study of bacteremia among residents of a long-term care facility, Muder et al [35] reported that infected pressure ulcers were the second leading cause of bacteremia (following urinary tract infections) and the most likely source of polymicrobial bacteremia. Less common soft tissue infections occasionally resulting from chronic wounds include necrotizing fasciitis, gas gangrene, and local abscess formation [36,37].

Osteomyelitis clearly is the most difficult infection to diagnose and treat in patients with chronic wounds. Its frequency has been estimated to be 17% to 25% in the setting of a nonhealing pressure ulcer and 38% in patients who have infected pressure ulcers [38–40]. Clinical signs suggestive of underlying osteomyelitis include bone exposure on direct examination and failure of wound closure (or its reopening) despite removal of pressure from the ulcer [41,42]. A recent review [43] highlights this point by recommending evaluation for osteomyelitis if a clean full thickness pressure ulcer has not improved after 4 weeks of treatment. Confirming the diagnosis is difficult. The most reliable method is by bone biopsy obtained before antibiotic administration (or 2 weeks after antibiotics have been discontinued) for histopathology as well as aerobic and anaerobic culture. The histopatholgic examination showing acute or chronic inflammatory changes of osteomyelitis is crucial to confirm the diagnosis. In addition, bone culture is necessary to choose the best antibiotic treatment program to be delivered over a period of at least 6 weeks [38,41]. Unfortunately, all other currently available methods of examination such as plain radiography, computed tomography, magnetic resonance imaging (MRI) and radionuclide scintigraphy yield results that are either too nonspecific or insensitive, with the possible exception of MRI. This relatively new technology needs more study to better assess its reliability in diagnosing osteomyelitis in the setting of a pressure ulcer [44].

The types of organisms causing osteomyelitis, similar to those causing self-tissue infections of the skin, subcutaneous tissue, fascia, or muscle, are usually multiple, especially when osteomyelitis involves bones of the pelvis or sacrum where fecal soilage is common. Typical organisms include S. aureus, streptococci, anaerobes, and gram-negative bacilli [41].

Infections of skin graft and tissue flaps

The last of the three major consequences of microorganisms within chronic wounds is the failure of surgical closure of large, slowly healing ulcers. Closure usually is attempted by direct closure or by skin grafts or the mobilization of large composite soft tissue flaps. An inherent risk with such a procedure is the potential for microorganisms colonizing the ulcer bed to proliferate after being enclosed and ultimately to destroy the graft. Garg et al [42] reported a 2.5% to 8% infection rate following myocutaneous flap surgery in spinal injury patients. Quantitative bacterial culture of tissue obtained from the ulcer bed before surgery is recommended by several investigators. Wound closure should be postponed until there are less than 10^5 organisms/g of tissue and no β-hemolytic streptococci present [22].

Clinical approach to patients with chronic wounds

Many excellent reviews and practice guidelines focusing on the management of chronic wounds recently have been published [18,43,45–48]. All agree that there is no place for routine cultures obtained by swab, aspiration, or tissue biopsy of wounds that are clinically uninfected. In addition, there is widespread agreement that systemic antibiotics are not indicated in patients with chronic, stable, uninfected wounds.

Presently, there is insufficient evidence to confirm or reject the hypothesis that microorganisms (by means of high colony count, presence of specific organisms or combination of organisms, or subclinical inflammatory response) cause or contribute to delayed healing of clinically uninfected ulcers. Because this question remains open and in need of further well-designed clinical trials, controversy regarding culture and use of topical antimicrobial agents continues to focus on this area of management. Until more reliable data are available, this author believes that emphasis on managing slowly healing, clinically uninfected chronic wounds should be placed on well-supported interventions, reviewed elsewhere in this issue. Consideration of tissue biopsy for quantitative microbiology and directed topical antimicrobial therapy as a time-limited therapeutic trial might be given only for cases that fail to respond. Management of clinical infections, such as cellulitis, sepsis, or osteomyelitis, generally is not a point of contention. Topical antimicrobial agents may be used for early, localized cellulitis, whereas systemic antibiotics chosen in accordance with wound, blood, or bone cultures are recommended for more serious soft tissue infection, sepsis, or osteomyelitis.

The preferred method of obtaining cultures from chronic, infected wounds is more variable in clinical practice and in recent reviews. Nevertheless, there is a general consensus that single swab cultures taken from the wound surface are least desirable because they do not reliably reflect the microorganisms invading tissue. Rather, more reliable techniques include quantitative cultures of samples obtained by tissue biopsy, needle aspiration, or possibly by "quantitative swab technique" [13,44,49].

Finally, most reviewers support the practice of obtaining tissue biopsy of the ulcer base for quantitative microbiology before performing ulcer closure procedures such as skin grafting, flap closure, or direct closure. The failure rate of these procedures is increased if greater than 10^5 organisms/g of tissue is obtained before surgery. In those circumstances, a systemic or topical course of antibiotics over several days to reduce the population density before closure is probably indicated [42,50].

Summary

- Chronic pressure ulcers and leg ulcers are common, especially in the elderly, and are a source of much distress and disability. Health care providers must distinguish between clinically unimportant but predictable colonization of these wounds and clinically relevant infection. Infection may present as increased local pain, cellulitis, local abscess, necrotizing fasciitis, osteomyelitis, bacteremia, or sepsis. For most of these conditions, systemic antibiotics are necessary.

- The use of topical antimicrobial agents as a means of promoting healing in clinically uninfected wounds is a subject of active investigation at this time. Currently, evidence is insufficient to support routine use of antimicrobial agents for this purpose.

- A quantitative tissue culture taken from the ulcer bed, revealing greater than 10^5 organisms/g of tissue appears to increase the risk of failure of ulcer wound closure by graft or flap. A short course of topical or systemic antibiotics before surgery in these instances is advisable.

References

[1] Lyder CH. Pressure ulcer prevention and management. JAMA 2003;289(2):223–6.
[2] Hansson C, Andersson E, Swanbeck G. Leg ulcer epidemiology in Gothenburg. Acta Chir Scand 1988;544(Suppl):S12–6.
[3] Sopata M, Luczak J, Ciupinska M. Effect of bacteriological status on pressure ulcer healing in patients with advanced cancer. J Wound Care 2002;11(3):107–10.
[4] Stephens P, Wall IB, Wilson MJ, et al. Anaerobic cocci populating the deep tissues of chronic wounds impair cellular wound healing responses in vitro. Br J Dermatol 2003;148(3):456–66.
[5] Sapico FL, Ginunas VJ, Thornhill-Joynes M, et al. Quantitative microbiology of pressure sores in different stages of healing. Diagn Microbiol Infect Dis 1986;5(1):31–8.
[6] Chow AW, Galpin JE, Guze LB. Clindamycin for treatment of sepsis caused by decubitus ulcers. J Infect Dis 1977;135(Suppl):S65–8.
[7] Hansson C, Hoborn J, Moller A, et al. The microbial flora in venous leg ulcers without clinical signs of infection: repeated culture using a validated standardized microbiological technique. Acta Derm Venereol 1995;75(1):24–30.
[8] Bowler PG, Davies BJ. The microbiology of infected and noninfected leg ulcers. Int J Dermatol 1999;38(8):573–8.
[9] Brook I, Frazier EH. Aerobic and anaerobic microbiology of chronic venous ulcers. Int J Dermatol 1998;37(6):426–8.
[10] Halbert AR, Stacey MC, Rohr JB, et al. The effect of bacterial colonization on venous ulcer healing. Australas J Dermatol 1992;33(2):75–80.
[11] Murdoch DA, Mitchelmore IJ, Tabaqchali S. The clinical importance of gram-positive anaerobic cocci isolated at St Bartholomew's Hospital, London, in 1987. J Med Microbiol 1994;41(1):36–44.
[12] Hill KE, Davies CE, Wilson MJ, et al. Molecular analysis of the microflora in chronic venous leg ulceration. J Med Microbiol 2003;52:365–9.
[13] Kunimoto BT. Assessment of venous leg ulcers: an in-depth discussion of a literature-guided approach. Ostomy Wound Manage 2001;47(5):38–49.
[14] Cutting KF, Harding KG. Criteria for identifying wound infection. J Wound Care 1994;3: 198–201.
[15] Lindholm C. Pressure ulcers and infection–understanding clinical features. Ostomy Wound Manage 2003;49(Suppl):S4–7.
[16] Clyne CA, Ramsden WH, Chant AD, et al. Oxygen tension on the skin of the gaiter area of limbs with venous disease. Br J Surg 1985;72(8):644–7.
[17] Burnand KG, Whimster I, Naidoo A, et al. Pericapillary fibrin in the ulcer-bearing skin of the leg: the cause of lipodermatosclerosis and venous ulceration. BMJ 1982;295:1071–2.

[18] Thomas DR. Issues and dilemmas in the prevention and treatment of pressure ulcers: a review. J Gerontol A Biol Sci Med 2001;56(6):M328–40.

[19] Trengove NJ, Stacey MC, McGechie DF, et al. Qualitative bacteriology and leg ulcer healing. J Wound Care 1996;5(6):277–80.

[20] Schmidtchen A, Holst E, Tapper H, et al. Elastase-producing *Pseudomonas aeruginosa* degrade plasma proteins and extracellular products of human skin and fibroblasts, and inhibit fibroblast growth. Microb Pathog 2003;34(1):47–55.

[21] Schmidtchen A, Wolff H, Hansson C. Differential proteinase expression by *Pseudomonas aeruginosa* derived from chronic leg ulcers. Acta Derm Venereol 2001;81(6):406–9.

[22] Heggers JP. Assessing and controlling wound infection. Clin Plast Surg 2003;30(1):25–35.

[23] Elek SD. Experimental staphylococcal infections in the skin of man. Ann N Y Acad Sci 1956; 65(3):85–90.

[24] Kass EH. Bacteriuria and the diagnosis of infections of the urinary tract; with observations on the use of methionine as a urinary antiseptic. Arch Intern Med 1957;100(5):709–14.

[25] Lindberg RB, Moncrief JA, Switzer WE, et al. The successful control of burn wound sepsis. J Trauma 1965;5(5):601–16.

[26] Teplitz C, Davis D, Mason AD Jr, et al. Pseudomonas burn wound sepsis. I pathogenesis of experimental pseudomonas burn wound sepsis. J Surg Res 1964;54:200–16.

[27] Bendy RH Jr, Nuccio PA, Wolfe E, et al. Relationship of quantitative wound bacterial counts to healing of decubiti: effect of topical gentamicin. Antimicrob Agents Chemother 1964;10:147–55.

[28] Robson MC. Wound infection. A failure of wound healing caused by an imbalance of bacteria. Surg Clin North Am 1997;7(3):637–50.

[29] Davies CE, Wilson MJ, Hill KE, et al. Use of molecular techniques to study microbial diversity in the skin: chronic wounds reevaluated. Wound Repair Regen 2001;9(5):332–40.

[30] Trengove NJ, Bielefeldt-Ohmann H, Stacey MC. Mitogenic activity and cytokine levels in non-healing and healing chronic leg ulcers. Wound Repair Regen 2000;8(1):13–25.

[31] Bryan CS, Dew CE, Reynolds KL. Bacteremia associated with decubitus ulcers. Arch Intern Med 1983;43(11):2093–5.

[32] Galpin JE, Chow AW, Bayer AS, et al. Sepsis associated with decubitus ulcers. Am J Med 1976;61(3):346–50.

[33] Colsky AS, Kirsner RS, Kerdel FA. Analysis of antibiotic susceptibilities of skin wound flora in hospitalized dermatology patients: the crisis of antibiotic resistance has come to the surface. Arch Dermatol 1998;134(8):1006–9.

[34] Robson MC, Heggers JP. Surgical infection. II: the beta-hemolytic streptococcus. J Surg Res 1969;9(5):289–92.

[35] Muder RR, Brennen C, Wagener MM, et al. Bacteremia in a long-term-care facility: a five-year prospective study of 163 consecutive episodes. Clin Infect Dis 1992;14(3):647–54.

[36] Kaplan LJ, Pameijer C, Blank-Reid C, et al. Necrotizing fasciitis: an uncommon consequence of pressure ulceration. Adv Wound Care 1998;11(4):185–9.

[37] Shibuya H, Terashi H, Kurata S, et al. Gas gangrene following sacral pressure sores. J Dermatol 1994;21(7):518–23.

[38] Darouiche RO, Landon GC, Klima M, et al. Osteomyelitis associated with pressure sores. Arch Intern Med 1994;154(7):753–8.

[39] Agency for Health Care Policy and Research. Pressure ulcer treatment: clinical practice guidelines. Washington (DC): Government Printing Office; 1994.

[40] Sugarman B, Hawes S, Musher DM, et al. Osteomyelitis beneath pressure sores. Arch Intern Med 1983;43(4):683–8.

[41] Sugarman B. Pressure sores and underlying bone infection. Arch Intern Med 1987;147(3): 553–5.

[42] Garg M, Rubayi S, Montgomerie JZ. Postoperative wound infections following myocutaneous flap surgery in spinal injury patients. Paraplegia 1992;30(10):734–9.

[43] Bates-Jensen BM. Quality indicators for prevention and management of pressure ulcers in vulnerable elders. Ann Intern Med 2001;135(8):744–51.

[44] Livesley NJ, Chow AW. Infected pressure ulcers in elderly individuals. Clin Infect Dis 2002; 35(11):1390–6.

[45] Walker P. Management of pressure ulcers. Oncology 2001;15(11):1499–508.

[46] O'Meara SM, Cullum NA, Majid M, et al. Systematic review of antimicrobial agents used for chronic wounds. Br J Surg 2001;88(1):4–21.

[47] Harper D, Gilles T, Anderson L, et al. Scottish Intercollegiate Guidelines Network. The care of patients with chronic leg ulcer. number 26. Edinburgh: SIGN Publication; 1998. p. 1–21.

[48] O'Meara S, Cullum N, Majid M, et al. Systematic reviews of wound care management: (3) antimicrobial agents for chronic wounds; (4) diabetic foot ulceration. number 21. Southampton (UK): The National Coordinating Centre for Health Technology Assessment; 2000. p. 1–237.

[49] Stotts NA. Determination of bacterial burden in wounds. Adv Wound Care 1995;8(4):46–52.

[50] Montgomerie JZ. Infections in patients with spinal cord injuries. Clin Infect Dis 1997;25(6): 1285–90.

ELSEVIER
SAUNDERS

NURSING
CLINICS
OF NORTH AMERICA

Nurs Clin N Am 40 (2005) 217–231

Dressings and More: Guidelines for Topical Wound Management

Dorothy Doughty, MN, RN, CWOCN, FAAN

Emory University Wound Ostomy Continence Nursing Education Center,
Room AT 732, 1365 Clifton Road, NE, Atlanta, GA 30322, USA

Because we have learned more about the wound healing process, it has become increasingly clear that topical therapy is only one aspect of effective wound care; it is equally important to correct the causative and contributing factors of a wound and to address the systemic factors that are critical to repair [1]. However, topical therapy does play an important role; dressings and other topical agents contribute to repair by eliminating known impediments to repair and by creating an environment favorable to the healing process [1–3]. We now know a lot more about what constitutes an optimal environment for repair, and we have an ever-increasing array of topical therapies designed to support wound healing. Most of the dressings and topical agents currently available provide passive support for wound healing, but there are an increasing number of therapies designed to actively manipulate the repair process. This article focuses on principle- and evidence-based topical therapy.

Principles of topical therapy

Wound healing requires the synthesis of connective tissue by fibroblasts and the formation of a new covering of epithelium by keratinocytes [4,5]. The goal in providing topical therapy is to eliminate impediments to fibroblast and keratinocyte activity and to maintain an environment that supports collagen synthesis and epithelial migration. Specifically, this goal involves the elimination of necrotic tissue, control of bacterial loads, management of wound exudate, maintenance of open proliferative wound edges, and provision of a moist, insulated, and protected wound surface (Box 1) [1–3,5].

E-mail address: ddought@emory.edu

0029-6465/05/$ - see front matter © 2005 Elsevier Inc. All rights reserved.
doi:10.1016/j.cnur.2004.09.012   *nursing.theclinics.com*

Box 1. Principles of topical therapy

Remove impediments to repair
- Debride necrotic tissue
- Identify and treat infection
- Wick and absorb exudate
- Eliminate trauma to wound bed

Maintain an environment conducive to repair
- Maintain moist wound surface
- Maintain open wound edges
- Insulate wound
- Provide bacterial barrier if needed (to prevent bacterial invasion)

Debridement

Necrotic tissue is a known impediment to the repair process and an optimum medium for bacterial growth; thus, debridement is an important initial goal whenever the goal is repair or the wound is infected [6,7]. Once the decision has been made to debride the wound, the clinician must make a decision regarding the approach to debridement. Options include surgical or instrumental removal of necrotic tissue, the use of enzymatic ointments to separate nonviable from viable tissue, Dakin's solution-soaked gauze dressings to help dissolve the necrotic tissue, and moisture-retentive dressings to promote autolysis (breakdown of the necrotic tissue by the white blood cells and enzymes in the wound fluid) [6,7].

Control of bacterial loads

Open wounds are always populated by bacteria, and infection is a well-established impediment to repair. Studies [2,8,9] have shown that wounds will not heal in the presence of invasive infection (ie, cellulitis or osteomyelitis) and that colony counts greater than 100,000 colony-forming units/mL will cause the failure of flaps and grafts in most cases. However, low levels of bacteria have been shown to actually stimulate repair. Thus, the critical question in terms of bacterial load seems to be: how many colony-forming units are too many, that is, at what point is treatment required to reduce the bioburden? Current clinical wisdom suggests that treatment is required for clinical infection (ie, invasion of the surrounding tissue as evidenced by cellulitis or osteomyelitis) and for evidence of bacterial loads sufficient to interfere with the repair process, a condition that has been called "critical colonization" [2,8–10]. Clinical indicators that the bacterial burden is compromising repair include poor quality granulation tissue, sudden "thinning" of granulation tissue, an increased volume of exudate, increased pain, and recurrent formation of an adherent layer of fibrinous slough [9].

A second question to be addressed is: what is the role of topical therapy in the management of bacterial loads? Although there are insufficient data to provide a definitive answer, there is general agreement that invasive infection requires systemic antibiotic therapy as well as topical measures to reduce the bacterial burden [2,8,9]. When the adverse effects of the bacterial loads are confined to the wound surface and the repair process, treatment usually involves primarily topical therapy, with systemic therapy reserved for particularly vulnerable patients and those who fail to respond to topical therapy. The third question then becomes: what are the guidelines and options for topical therapy to reduce bacterial loads? Local measures to control bacterial loads include routine cleansing to mechanically "flush" bacteria and toxins from the wound surface and the use of antiseptic agents, antimicrobial dressings, and topical antibiotics to kill bacteria at the wound surface (Table 1) [2,9,11]. The following are specific guidelines and considerations for controlling bacterial loads.

Cleansing

Effective wound cleansing is an important element of care for any wound with necrotic tissue or a large volume of exudate. The goal is to mechanically flush nonviable tissue, bacteria, and bacterial toxins from the wound surface without damaging the viable tissue or driving the bacteria into the underlying tissue. Studies [2,9] performed to date indicate that the optimal level of irrigation force is 5 to 15 psi; a lower pressure is ineffective in dislodging bacteria from the wound surface, and a higher pressure may cause bacterial penetration or damage to the underlying tissue. Effective cleansing methods include the use of a 35-cc syringe with an 18-gauge angiographic catheter, commercial wound cleansing devices designed to provide 5 to 15 psi irrigating force, wound cleansers packaged in vacuum systems that deliver the desired amount of pressure, and pulsatile lavage systems, which provide effective irrigation force along with concurrent removal of the irrigant by suction. The force of the irrigating stream seems to be more critical than the type of solution used, although further studies are needed. Saline and tap water (including showering for ambulatory patients) are the most commonly used cleansers, although commercial cleansers packaged with a preservative to assure long-term sterility are beneficial in long-term and home care settings [2,9].

Antiseptic agents

The use of antiseptics remains one of the major controversies in wound care. Although there is consensus that antiseptics are damaging to fibroblasts and therefore contraindicated in granulating wounds, the role of antiseptics in the management of infected wounds is less clear [2,9,12,13]. A reasonable approach at present is to limit the use of antiseptic agents to wounds with evidence of a heavy bioburden, to use agents and dilutions that minimize any adverse effects, and to discontinue antiseptics as soon as

Table 1
Antibacterial agents

Product	Beneficial effects	Considerations
Cleanser Technicare (chloroxylenol and cocamidopropyl PG-dimonium chloride) (CareTech Laboratories)	Broad spectrum bactericidal with minimum cytotoxicity; residual antibacterial effects persist for 24 hours	Apply to wound for 2 minutes then rinse thoroughly (do not pack wound with cleanser)
Antiseptic Dakin's solution (sodium hypochlorite) 0.025% (concentration with minimal cytotoxic effects)	Broad spectrum bactericidal effects; promotes dissolution of necrotic tissue; provides odor control	Limit use to infected necrotic wounds; avoid exposure to heat and light (inactivates product); requires changing dressing twice daily
Antibacterial dressings Cadexomer iodine Iodosorb and Iodoflex (Healthpoint, Ft Worth, TX)	Gradual release of iodine provides sustained antibacterial effects and prevents damage to good cells	Minor stinging occurs in small percentage of patients; avoid use on large surfaces and in patients with iodine allergy
Sustained release silver dressings	Gradual release of silver provides broad spectrum bactericidal activity with no damage to good cells and no apparent development of bacterial resistance	Available in multiple forms; absorbers: Acticoat (Smith and Nephew, Largo, FL); Silvasorb (Medline, Mundelein IL); Actisorb (Johnson & Johnson, Arlington TX); Contreet Coloplast, Marietta GA) Contact layer: Silverlon (Argentum, Lakemont GA) Hydraters: Silvasorb Gel (Medline, Mundeline, IL)

bacterial balance has been restored, as evidenced by a clean wound bed and a reduced volume of exudate.

Antimicrobial dressings

One of the most exciting advances in topical therapy has been the development of sustained release antimicrobial dressings. These dressings are impregnated with antiseptic agents (either cadexomer iodine or ionic silver) that kill bacteria on the wound surface or within the dressing for as long as 7 days. Both iodine and silver provide a broad antibacterial spectrum, and neither has been associated with toxicity to fibroblasts or newly formed connective tissues; thus they seem to be the ideal agents for wounds with evidence of heavy bioburden [14–18]. However, there are many questions yet to be answered in regard to the optimal use of these agents; for example, some of the silver agents are designed to be surface active, that is, they kill bacteria on the wound surface, whereas other agents are designed to kill the bacteria within the dressing matrix. It is not yet known whether there are clinical advantages to either approach. Among the silver-based dressings there are also differences in the rate at which the ionic silver is released, with some dressings providing an initial bolus and others providing a steady release; again, data are currently lacking to make recommendations regarding an optimal approach. Presently, clinicians generally select a particular agent based on wound characteristics and frequency of dressing change [3].

Topical antibiotics

Topical antibiotics may be used alone or in conjunction with systemic antibiotics to eliminate known pathogens; for example, mupirocin (Bactroban) is sometimes used to treat methicillin-resistant *Staphylococcus aureus* [14]. Appropriate use of topical antibiotics requires a wound culture and sensitivity to identify the specific pathogen and agents to which it is responsive.

Osteomyelitis, cellulitis, and impaired wound healing are all potential complications of chronic wounds caused by excessive bacterial loads. Therefore, effective management of any open wound should include appropriate cleansing, ongoing monitoring for evidence of infectious complications, and prompt interventions to restore bacterial balance [2,9,14].

Establishment of open wound edges

Repair of open wounds culminates with the establishment of a new epithelial covering, which involves the migration of epithelial cells from the wound edges. Epithelial migration cannot occur when the wound edges are sealed with mature epithelium, a condition also known as "epibole" [1,5,19]. In this situation, the clinician must reestablish an open wound edge, that is, by exposure of the reproducing, advancing edge of the epidermis (Fig. 1 shows closed versus open wound edges). In some situations this can be accomplished by repetitive cauterization of the wound edges with $AgNO_3$ to eliminate the covering epithelium; however, when this is not effective, surgical excision is indicated [1,5,19]. Cauterization of the covering epithelium is sometimes painful, so the clinician should always monitor the patient closely for any discomfort and should use topical analgesics when indicated.

Exudate management

Effective exudate management is a critical element of topical therapy. Studies [1,5,20] indicate that chronic wound fluid contains high levels of

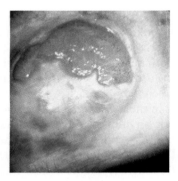

Fig. 1. Open versus closed wound edges. Note the open proliferative wound edges on the inferior aspect of the wound compared with the closed wound edges on the superior aspect of the wound.

inflammatory mediators that adversely affect wound repair; thus, the topical therapy program must include measures to effectively wick exudate from tunneled and undermined areas and to prevent pooling of exudate on the wound surface. There are a number of dressings on the market that can be used to appropriately manage exudate. The most commonly used absorptive dressings include alginates, hydrofibers, foams and related dressings, absorptive powders, and gauze. These agents may be used alone or in combination to minimize the amount of exudate in contact with the wound surface; most are designed to be changed daily or every other day [1–3,18,21]. The frequency of dressing change is determined by the volume of exudate and any conditions that mandate more frequent wound assessment, such as wound infection. Gauze deserves special mention, because it is the most commonly used and yet the least effective option. Gauze dressings provide limited absorption, require much more frequent dressing changes, cause cooling of the wound bed, and are the dressing material most likely to be incorrectly used (overpacking and traumatic removal of dry gauze dressings are common adverse effects of gauze dressings) [1,3,22]. Table 2 provides examples of absorptive dressings.

Maintenance moist wound surface

Winter's research [23] clearly established the beneficial effects of a moist wound surface in the repair process. A moist wound surface promotes cell migration and prevents cell death. The standard of care in topical therapy is now "moist wound healing," which means that all wounds should be managed with dressings and products that prevent desiccation of the wound surface. In caring for wounds with minimal or no exudate, the clinician must select agents that maintain or donate moisture at the wound surface [1–3,18]. The most commonly used types of hydrating dressings are hydrogels,

Table 2
Commonly used dressings

Dressing type	Examples
Absorptive dressings	
Calcium alginates (rope and flat)	Kaltostat (ConvaTec, Princeton NJ); AlgiSite (Smith & Nephew, Largo, FL); Tegagen (3M, St. Paul, MN)
Hydrofibers (rope and flat)	Aquacel, Aquacel Ag (ConvaTec)
Foams and polymer dressings (usually flat cover dressings)	Allevyn (Smith & Nephew, Largo, FL); Tielle (Johnson & Johnson, Arlington TX); Mepilex (Molnlycke, Newtown PA); Biatain, Contreet (Coloplast, Marietta GA); Versiva (ConvaTec, Princeton NJ)
Hypertonic saline gauze	Mesalt (Molnlycke, Newtown PA)
Hydrating dressings	
Gels	
Amorphous	Curasol (Healthpoint, Ft Worth TX); Carrasyn (Carrington, Irving TX)
Solid	Dermal gel (glycerine-based gel sheet) (Medline, Mundelein IL)
Hydrocolloids	DuoDERM (ConvaTec, Princeton NJ); Tegasorb (3M, St. Paul, MN)
Transparent adhesive dressings	OpSite (Smith & Nephew, Largo FL); Tegaderm (3 M, St. Paul, MN)
Nonadherent gauze	Adaptic (Johnson & Johnson, TX); Mepitel (Molnlycke, Newtown PA)

hydrocolloids, transparent adhesive dressings, and nonadherent gauze dressings (see Table 2) [1–3,18]. The frequency of dressing change varies from several times daily to 1 to 2 times per week, depending on the amount of moisture within the wound and the ability of the dressing to maintain a moist surface and prevent both desiccation and overhydration. Again, gauze is usually the least appropriate choice because it requires frequent dressing changes, is prone to rapid dehydration and traumatic removal, and provides no bacterial barrier [1,3,22].

Maintenance protected insulated wound surface

The optimal wound environment is one that is protected from bacterial invasion, surface trauma, and hypothermia. The clinician should select a dressing that provides a bacterial barrier, atraumatic removal, and insulation, whenever possible. All moisture-retentive dressings provide atraumatic removal as long as they are changed frequently enough to prevent desiccation of the wound surface. Foam, hydrocolloid, and transparent adhesive dressings provide insulation as well as a bacterial barrier and are therefore good choices for cover dressings [1–3].

Guidelines for dressing selection

In selecting dressings for a particular wound, the goal is to match dressing characteristics to wound characteristics and needs. Generally, dressings can be classified as filler or cover dressings. Filler dressings are available in amorphous and rope forms and are designed to be placed into wounds with depth or dead space, whereas cover dressings are flat dressings intended to be placed over wounds. Dressings can also be classified as absorptive or hydrating, as noted above [1–3].

Wound characteristics to be considered when selecting dressings include the wound depth, presence of dead space (ie, undermined or tunneled areas), volume of exudate, and the need for a bacterial barrier, which is determined by wound location and presence of contaminants such as urine and stool. Selection of the primary dressing (wound contact layer) is based on the wound depth, presence of tunnels or undermined areas, and volume of exudate. The selection of the cover dressing is based on the volume of exudate and the need for a bacterial barrier [1–3]. Based on these principles, wounds can be classified as deep wet wounds, deep dry wounds, shallow wet wounds, or shallow dry wounds (Table 3).

Deep wet wounds

Deep wet wounds are characterized by a depth greater than 0.5 cm or tunneled and undermined areas, and moderate to large amounts of exudate. These wounds require an absorptive filler dressing plus an absorptive cover dressing (Fig. 2). Options for the absorptive filler include an alginate, hydrofiber, or foam in rope form, absorptive gel strands, or damp gauze. If the wound is associated with a narrow tunnel (ie, a tunnel ≤0.2 cm in diameter), a ribbon gauze strip can be used to wick exudate from the tunnel without risking overpacking of the tunnel. (Excessive packing creates a pressure dressing effect and compromises the wound's ability to close.) Good choices for ribbon gauze include NuGauze (Johnson & Johnson, Arlington, TX) and Mesalt Rope (Molnlycke Health care, Newtown, PA), a ribbon form gauze impregnated with hypertonic saline. Options for an absorptive cover dressing include an adhesive foam dressing or gauze and tape combination. If the wound is on the extremity, gauze or nonadhesive foam secured with wrap gauze is another option. For trunk wounds in incontinent patients, the cover dressing must provide an effective bacterial barrier, for example, an adhesive waterproof foam dressing or a gauze cover dressing with waterproof tape or transparent adhesive dressing cover.

Deep dry wounds

Deep dry wounds are more than 0.5 cm deep or show tunneled and undermined areas and have minimal or no exudate. These wounds require a hydrating filler dressing plus a hydrating cover dressing (Fig. 3) and are most effectively managed with a layer of amorphous gel followed by loosely

Table 3
Guidelines for dressing selection

Classify the wound
    Wounds with depth ≥0.5 cm, tunnels, or undermined areas and moderate to large
      volumes of exudate = deep and wet
    Wounds with depth ≥0.5 cm, tunnels, or undermined areas and minimal or no
      exudate = deep and dry
    Wounds ≤0.5 cm deep with no tunnels or undermined areas and moderate to large
      volumes of exudate = shallow and wet
    Wounds ≤0.5 cm deep with no tunnels or undermined areas and minimal or no
      exudate = shallow and dry

Select Dressing Option

Deep wet wounds	Deep dry wounds
Filler Dressing Options	Filler Dressing Options
Calcium alginate (flat or rope)	Liquid gel plus lightly fluffed damp gauze
Hydrofiber (flat or rope)	Gel-soaked gauze fluffed into wound
Hypertonic saline gauze (flat or rope)	Cover Dressing Options
Damp gauze fluffed into wound	Gauze plus transparent adhesive dressing[a]
Cover Dressing Options	Waterproof adhesive foam dressing[a]
Gauze plus tape	
Gauze plus transparent adhesive dressing[a]	
Waterproof adhesive foam dressing[a]	

Shallow wet wounds	Shallow dry wounds
Foam dressing with adhesive border[a]	Solid hydrogel with adhesive border[a];
Alginate plus adhesive foam[a]; alginate	solid hydrogel plus wrap gauze
plus wrap gauze	Hydrocolloid[a]
Hydrofiber plus adhesive foam[a];	Nonadherent gauze + gauze cover
hydrofiber plus wrap gauze	Transparent adhesive dressing[a]
Nonadherent gauze plus gauze cover	

    [a] Provides bacterial barrier.

fluffed damp gauze. Gel-soaked ribbon gauze (eg, NuGauze) is available for narrow tunnels. Options for cover dressings include gauze secured by a transparent adhesive dressing, an adhesive foam dressing, or a gauze and tape combination; for extremity wounds the gauze can be secured with wrap gauze.

Shallow wet wounds

    Shallow wet wounds show a depth less than 0.5 cm, no tunneled or undermined areas, and moderate to large amounts of exudate. These wounds require an absorptive cover dressing (Fig. 4). (A contact layer is optional with these wounds but may be used to add absorptive capacity.) Good dressing choices include flat alginate or hydrofiber dressings with a foam or gauze cover, a nonadherent contact layer such as Adaptic (Johnson & Johnson, Arlington, TX) plus a foam or gauze cover, and adhesive foam dressings alone. Hydrocolloid dressings (eg, Duoderm, ConvaTec, Princeton, NJ) have frequently been used for these wounds in the

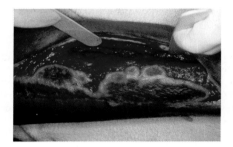

Fig. 2. Deep wet wound. The wound shows extensive undermining and a moderate amount of exudate. An absorptive filler type dressing such as calcium alginate or hydrofiber plus an absorptive cover (eg, gauze and wrap gauze or adhesive foam) is indicated. A bacterial barrier is not essential because this wound is located on an extremity.

past; however, maceration is a common problem because hydrocolloid dressings are designed to absorb limited amounts of exudate.

Shallow dry wounds

Shallow dry wounds are characterized by a depth less than 0.5 cm, no tunneled or undermined areas, and minimal or no exudate. These wounds require a hydrating cover dressing (a nonadherent contact layer may be used but is optional) (Fig. 5). Good dressing options for trunk wounds include hydrocolloid dressings, thin adhesive foam dressings, and transparent adhesive dressings; options for extremity wounds include solid gel dressings or nonadherent contact layers (eg, Adaptic) in combination with gauze and wrap gauze. Solid gel dressings are available in water- and glycerin-based formulations. Glycerin-based products are advantageous because they resist dehydration and can absorb minimal to moderate amounts of exudate. Shallow wounds in difficult-to-dress areas such as the gluteal fold may be managed with an absorptive skin barrier paste (eg, a zinc oxide-based moisture barrier product) that absorbs drainage and maintains a moist

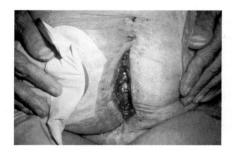

Fig. 3. Deep dry wound. This wound shows a dehisced incision with a low volume of exudate. A hydrating filler type dressing, such as amorphous gel plus fluffed saline gauze and hydrating cover such as transparent adhesive dressing is required.

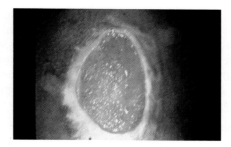

Fig. 4. Shallow wet wound. A wound with minimal depth, no undermining or tunneling, and a moderate amount of exudate requires an absorptive cover dressing such as adhesive foam (located on the trunk of an incontinent patient, so bacterial barrier is important).

surface; a folded gauze sponge may be tucked between the buttocks to reduce frictional forces.

Active wound therapies: indications and guidelines

All of the principles and products discussed thus far provide passive support for wound healing by providing absorption of exudate, maintaining a moist wound surface, and preventing or reducing bacterial contamination. When coupled with a comprehensive management program that also addresses causative factors and systemic support for wound repair, this level of support is usually all that is needed to promote healing. However, there is a subset of wounds that are refractory to standard care, as evidenced by the absence of measurable progress for 2 to 4 weeks despite appropriate comprehensive management. The reason for this failure to respond is believed to be some imbalance in the mixture of cellular-level substances that regulate wound repair (ie, growth factors, cytokines such as nitric

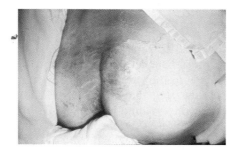

Fig. 5. Shallow dry wound. This is a wound with no depth or tunnels and minimal exudate. This type of wound requires a hydrating cover dressing with a bacterial barrier (because of location). Hydrocolloid is one good option.

oxide, matrix metalloproteinases, and others) [24,25]. Although we currently lack the diagnostic tools to determine the specific imbalance, we do now have access to a number of therapies that are designed to actively manipulate and stimulate the repair process; these therapies should be considered whenever a wound fails to respond to appropriate standard therapy. The most commonly used active wound therapies are highlighted below:

Matrix metalloproteinases inhibitors

Matrix metalloproteinases (MMP) are naturally occurring enzymes that play a beneficial role during the early phases of wound repair. However, persistent high levels of MMPs interfere with the proliferative phase of repair by binding the growth factors and breaking down the newly formed granulation tissue [5]. Promogran (Johnson & Johnson) is a new dressing that binds MMPs and therefore promotes growth factor activity and new tissue synthesis. Promogran is indicated for wounds that are clean but slow to granulate.

Topical growth factors

Growth factors are now recognized as the primary regulator of the repair process. Growth factors promote cell migration, stimulate cellular reproduction, and regulate specific processes critical to repair. Low levels of endogenous growth factors are believed to be one reason for the failure to heal, especially among diabetic patients, which has led to the production of products containing exogenous growth factors. Becaplermin (Regranex) is a gel that contains growth factors produced by recombinant DNA technology. It is indicated for use primarily for nonhealing ulcers in diabetic patients in conjunction with a comprehensive wound management program that must include offloading, elimination of infection, and tight glucose control [25,26]. Becaplermin is available only by prescription and costs $400 to $500 for a 15-g tube.

Negative pressure wound therapy

Negative pressure wound therapy (eg, VAC, KCI, San Antonio, TX) is currently one of the most beneficial active wound therapies. It involves placing a porous sponge into the wound bed followed by the application of a transparent adhesive dressing that seals the wound, and then applying a negative suction to the entire wound bed [3,25]. The results of the negative suction are effective elimination of the chronic wound fluid and activation of intracellular processes governing neoangiogenesis and granulation tissue formation. These beneficial effects are evidenced clinically by the rapid development of a well-vascularized wound bed and subsequent production of granulation tissue [3,25,27]. Negative pressure wound therapy is particularly effective for wounds that are viable but slow to granulate and deep wounds with a high volume of exudate and for the establishment of a well-vascularized wound bed in preparation for surgical closure and promotion of flap and graft survival. This therapy is contraindicated in wounds with exposed vessels and is generally considered inappropriate for necrotic and infected wounds. The cost of therapy is approximately $125 per day, so it is essential to use this therapy appropriately and to discontinue it once a healthy bed of granulation tissue has been established and the volume of exudate has diminished. At this point, treatment of the patient's wound can be safely crossed over to standard moist wound healing.

Electrical stimulation

The application of a high-voltage, pulsed current has been demonstrated in a number of studies [25,27,28] to promote wound repair and is specifically identified as an option for nonhealing wounds by the Agency for Health Care Policy and Research (now named the Agency for Healthcare Policy and Research) guidelines on pressure ulcers in adults. Typically, this therapy is provided by physical therapists, with a treatment frequency of once daily 5 to 7 times per week.

Monochromatic infrared energy

Monochromatic infrared energy is a relatively new option for nonhealing wounds (eg, Anodyne Therapy, Tampa, FL). It is approved for treatment of nonhealing wounds when compromised perfusion is believed to be the causative factor and is also approved for treatment of neuropathy [29,30]. This therapy involves the delivery of infrared energy to the wound bed, which reduces edema and causes the release of nitric oxide. The enhanced levels of nitric oxide improve arterial inflow (particularly the microcirculation) and promote venous return [30].

Human skin equivalents

Dermagraft is one type of dermal replacement that consists of a bioabsorbable mesh populated with newborn dermal fibroblasts and growth factors (eg, Dermagraft, Smith and Nephew, Largo, FL). The dermal mesh promotes granulation tissue formation by providing additional fibroblasts in addition to growth factors and is, therefore, indicated for wounds that are clean but not granulating or very slow to granulate [3]. It can be reapplied weekly for up to 8 weeks if needed. The cost is approximately $500 per application.

Apligraf is a bilayered skin substitute. The dermal layer is composed of bovine collagen populated with human fibroblasts (derived from neonatal foreskin), and the epidermal layer is composed of keratinocytes (also derived from neonatal foreskin) [3,31]. The advantage of using neonatal foreskin as the source for fibroblasts and keratinocytes is that this tissue lacks the human lymphocytic antigen, so rejection has not been an issue. The graft is a living skin substitute that is eventually infiltrated by area blood vessels and populated by host keratinocytes, which results in long-term durability. Apligraf is indicated in situations in which a split thickness skin graft would be used (eg, refractory venous ulcers with a viable wound base) [31]. The cost is approximately $1200 per application, so appropriate use is critical.

Summary

Principle-based topical therapy is a key element of effective wound care. Most products on the market provide passive support for wound healing by creating an environment favorable to repair (ie, clean, moist, insulated, and protected). There are also emerging therapies designed to actively manipulate the repair process. The clinician must make product decisions based on wound characteristics and response to treatment.

References

[1] Rolstad B, Ovington L, Harris A. Principles of wound management. In: Bryant R, editor. Acute and chronic wounds: nursing management. 2nd edition. St. Louis (MO): Mosby; 2000. p. 85–124.

[2] Ovington L. Wound management: cleansing agents and dressings. In: Morison M, editor. The prevention and treatment of pressure ulcers. London: Mosby; 2001. p. 135–54.

[3] Baranoski S, Ayello E. Wound treatment options. In: Baranoski S, Ayello E, editors. Wound care essentials: practice principles. Philadelphia: Lippincott Williams & Wilkins; 2004. p. 127–56.

[4] Jones V, Bale S, Harding K. Acute and chronic wound healing. In: Baranoski S, Ayello E, editors. Wound care essentials: practice principles. Philadelphia: Lippincott Williams & Wilkins; 2004. p. 61–78.

[5] Waldrop J, Doughty D. Wound healing physiology. In: Bryant R, editor. Acute and chronic wounds: nursing management. 2nd edition. St. Louis (MO): Mosby; 2000. p. 17–40.

[6] Ramundo J, Wells J. Debridement. In: Bryant R, editor. Acute and chronic wounds: nursing management. 2nd edition. St. Louis (MO): Mosby; 2000. p. 157–78.

[7] Ayello E, Baranoski S, Kerstein M, et al. Wound debridement. In: Baranoski S, Ayello E, editors. Wound care essentials: practice principles. Philadelphia: Lippincott Williams & Wilkins; 2004. p. 117–26.

[8] Davis S, Mertz P, Eaglstein W. The wound environment: implications from research studies for healing and infection. In: Krasner D, Rodeheaver G, Sibbald R, editors. Chronic wound care: a clinical source book for healthcare professionals. 3rd edition. Wayne (PA): HMP Com-Munications; 2001. p. 253–64.

[9] Gardner S, Frantz R. Wound bioburden. In: Baranoski S, Ayello E, editors. Wound care essentials: practice principles. Philadelphia: Lippincott Williams & Wilkins; 2004. p. 91–116.

[10] Kingsley A. The wound infection continuum and its application to clinical practice. Ostomy Wound Manage 2003;49(Suppl 7A):S1–7.

[11] Stotts N. Wound infection: diagnosis and management. In: Bryant R, editor. Acute and chronic wounds: nursing management. 2nd edition. St. Louis (MO): Mosby; 2000. p. 179–88.

[12] Doughty D. A rational approach to the use of topical antiseptics. J Wound Ostomy Continence Nurs 1994;21:224–31.

[13] Heggers J, Sazy J, Stenberg B, et al. Bactericidal and wound-healing properties of sodium hypochlorite solutions: the 1991 Lindberg award. J Burn Care Rehabil 1991;12:420–4.

[14] Sibbald R, Williamson D, Orsted H, et al. Preparing the wound bed—debridement, bacterial balance, and moisture balance. Ostomy Wound Manage 2000;46(11):14–35.

[15] Sundberg J, Meller R. A retrospective review of the use of cadexomer iodine in the treatment of chronic wounds. Wounds 1997;9(3):68–86.

[16] Ovington L. Nanocrystalline silver: where the old and familiar meets a new frontier. Wounds 2001;13(Suppl 2B):S4–10.

[17] Wright J, Hansen D, Burrell R. The comparative efficacy of two antimicrobial barrier dressings: in-vitro examination of two controlled release of silver dressings. Wounds 1998; 10(6):179–88.

[18] Campton-Johnston S, Wilson J. Infected wound management: advanced technologies, moisture-retentive dressings, and die-hard methods. Crit Care Nurs Q 2001;24(2):64–77.

[19] Stotts N. Assessing a patient with a pressure ulcer. In: Morison M, editor. The prevention and treatment of pressure ulcers. London: Mosby; 2001. p. 99–116.

[20] Staiano-Coico L, Higgins P, Schwartz S, et al. Wound fluids: a reflection of the state of healing. Ostomy Wound Manage 2000;46(Suppl 1A):S85–93.

[21] Lionelli G, Lawrence W. Wound dressings. Surg Clin North Am 2003;83(3):617–38.

[22] Ovington L. Hanging wet-to-dry dressings out to dry. Home Healthc Nurse 2001;19(8): 477–84.

[23] Winter G. Formation of the scab and the rate of epithelialization of superficial wounds in the skin of young domestic pigs. Nature 1962;193:293–4.

[24] Schultz G. Molecular regulation of wound healing. In: Bryant R, editor. Acute and chronic wounds: nursing management. 2nd edition. St. Louis (MO): Mosby; 2000. p. 413–30.

[25] Broussard C, Mendez-Eastman S, Frantz R. Adjuvant wound therapies. In: Bryant R, editor. Acute and chronic wounds: nursing management. 2nd edition. St. Louis (MO): Mosby; 2000. p. 431–54.

[26] Brissett A, Hom D. The effects of tissue sealants, platelet gels, and growth factors on wound healing. Curr Opin Otolaryngol Head Neck Surg 2003;11(4):245–50.

[27] Hess C, Howard M, Attinger C. A review of mechanical adjuncts in wound healing: hydrotherapy, ultrasound, negative pressure therapy, hyperbaric oxygen, and electrostimulation. Ann Plast Surg 2003;51(2):210–8.

[28] Agency for Health Care Policy and Research. Clinical practice guideline: pressure ulcer treatment. Rockville (MD): US Department of Health and Human Services; 1994.

[29] Horwitz L, Burke T, Carnegie D. Augmentation of wound healing using monochromatic infrared energy. Adv Wound Care 1999;12:35–40.

[30] Burke T. Five questions—and answers—about MIRE treatment. Adv Wound Care 2003; 16(7):369–71.

[31] Dolynchuk K, Hull P, Guenther L, et al. The role of Apligraf in the treatment of venous leg ulcers. Ostomy Wound Manage 1999;45(1):34–43.

ELSEVIER
SAUNDERS

NURSING
CLINICS
OF NORTH AMERICA

Nurs Clin N Am 40 (2005) 233–249

Wound Debridement: Therapeutic Options and Care Considerations

Janice M. Beitz, PhD, RN, CS, CNOR, CWOCN

*School of Nursing, La Salle University, 1900 West Olney Avenue,
Philadelphia, PA 19141, USA*

Although the topic of wound healing physiology and its critical components have been described for many years, a greater emphasis on preparation of the wound bed for optimal healing and health has pervaded the contemporary literature [1,2,3]. This scrutiny makes supreme sense in the context of acute and especially chronic wound healing. Necrotic tissue and other similar substances serve to impede or totally halt wound healing. A wound bed in need of debridement will not improve until this impediment is removed.

The importance of debridement has been known for centuries. Early descriptions of debridement date back to Hippocrates who described the deleterious effects of leaving necrotic tissue in wounds [4]. This article addresses the topic of wound debridement, including issues in the use of debridement, available methods, and nursing considerations associated with implementation. When available, evidence-based practice approaches and best practices will underpin the discussion.

Benefits of wound debridement

What is wound bed preparation and why is it integrally related to wound debridement? Falanga [1] defines wound bed preparation as the "global management of the wound to accelerate endogenous healing or to facilitate the effectiveness of other therapeutic measures." Wound debridement is only one component of this facilitative process. Wound bed preparation is really composed of four considerations that have been organized into the mnemonic device "TIME": *T*issue that is nonviable or deficient must be debrided. *I*nfection (or inflammation) must be reduced and managed. *M*oisture imbalance or exudate control must be addressed to avoid desiccation or

---

E-mail address: beitz@lasalle.edu

maceration. *E*pidermal margins (or edges) of the wound must be examined for nonadvancement. Nonmigration of epidermal cells may signify the need for other adjunctive therapies [5,6,7].

What purposes do wound debridement serve? The word itself provides a clue because debridement derives from the French (*débrider*) meaning "to unbridle" or remove a restraint [8]. The process of debridement is important for several crucial reasons: to enhance wound assessment, to decrease the potential for infection, to activate important cellular activity, and to remove physical barriers to healing (necrotic tissue).

The critical nature of quality wound assessment pervades the modern literature on wound care. Necrotic tissue prevents recognition of true wound depth, the presence of tunneling and undermining, and deep infected material. Provided adequate blood supply is present, necrotic tissue must be removed from any wound for optimal assessment.

Debridement helps to remove bacteria. Evidence suggests that significant numbers of bacteria in a wound will slow healing. When bacteria exceed 100,000 (10^5) bacteria/g of tissue, wound healing processes do not proceed normally [9]. It is unclear whether bacterial burden is a cause or consequence of impaired healing [10]; however, it is clear that necrotic matter in a wound encourages growth of anaerobic bacteria that are deleterious.

Debridement also helps to remove biofilms, which are theorized to slow wound healing. Biofilms are certain bacteria and other organisms that are covered with an extrapolysaccharide matrix. Biofilms are resistant to antibiotics and the normal immune systems of the host [11,12].

Debriding processes may also ameliorate senescent cells. These aged cells have significantly less protein production and proliferation abilities. Debridement acts to reduce the presence of these senescent cells so that younger, healthier cells are available for wound healing. In addition, necrotic tissue leads to the release of endotoxins that inhibit keratinocytes and fibroblast activity [12].

Another role of debridement is to remove the excess tissue that surrounds chronic wounds. Neuropathic ulcers are often associated with callus formation. Excision of the callus allows tissue-healing cells to proliferate, migrate, and ultimately heal [2,10]. Another benefit of debridement is its effect on growth factor activity. It is hypothesized that chronic wounds are lacking in these proteins or that they may be unavailable for wound healing processes because of binding to proteins present in the chronic wound [13,14]. Debridement releases activated platelets that promulgate various growth factors and cytokines [15].

Necrotic tissue may also act to "splint" a wound; the presence of necrotic tissue can prevent closure by inhibiting wound contraction processes [16]. Conversely, if a wound closes prematurely over necrotic material, it can lead to dead space and potential abscess formation [17].

The multiple beneficial components of debridement are critically important to optimal outcomes. If initial wound assessment is incorrect, for example, subsequent treatment will likely be problematic. A necrotic wound that is diagnosed as a pressure ulcer but is really pyoderma gangrenosum will not respond to pressure reduction but will respond to medication therapy (eg, steroids and debridement to follow as necessary). For some persons with pyoderma gangrenosum, debridement may actually worsen the inflammatory process [18].

The process of wound healing: barriers and facilitators

An appreciation of the importance of wound debridement is enhanced when the discussion in placed in the context of wound healing. It is especially compelling in light of wound healing in chronic wounds.

Normal wound healing (the kind associated with acute wounds) is ordinarily structured in phases. Although the phases are often discussed separately, in reality they overlap. The four phases include hemostasis, inflammation, proliferation, and remodeling. Hemostasis follows injury immediately, and the primary purpose is clot formation. A major cell present in this phase is the platelet. Inflammation targets removal of bacteria and debris and, secondarily, stimulation of cells critical for subsequent phases. The major cell of this phase is the macrophage. Proliferation is the phase in which new blood vessels grow so that granulation tissue will form. The major cells are fibroblasts and endothelial cells. In the final phase, collagen deposited in the scar strengthens tissue to improve tensile strength.

Chronic wounds do not heal in this orderly and efficient way. Rather, systemic and local factors impede normal phase progression. These chronic wounds have been called "stuck" or "stunned" wounds [19,20]. Barriers include systemic issues such as older (or very young) age, stress, malnutrition, poor tissue oxygenation, immune suppression, concomitant diseases like diabetes or cancer, medication therapy (steroids or chemotherapy), or irradiation. Local factors are also critically important, including poor perfusion, tissue edema, high bacterial burden, lack of wound moisture, use of cytotoxic agents, mechanical stressors, inappropriate wound care, and, pertinent to the current discussion, the presence of necrotic tissue. The last factor is of major importance [21]. It is not accidental that the first factor in the TIME mnemonic is tissue debridement. Nonviable or deficient tissue will impede further improvement because it will be impossible to halt infection, to keep the wound bed moisture balanced, and to help epidermal edges come together. Stated simply, gangrenous, necrotic, devitalized, and ischemic tissue need to be debrided.

Debridement is a salient component of facilitators to wound healing. These facilitators include good nutrition, wound protection, a moist wound environment, adequate oxygen supply, appropriate bioburden, and amelioration of the cause of the wound if possible. However, even in the presence of multiple facilitators, overcoming necrotic tissue in a wound bed is difficult [22].

Special role of wound bed debridement

The positive clinical outcome of wound debridement is a viable wound base. This viability allows for the correct functioning of growth factors and decreased inflammatory cytokines, proteases, and deleterious substances. Debridement should be distinguished from wound cleansing. Wound cleansing is used to remove foreign materials, reduce bioburden, and ameliorate odor and exudates. Topical cleansing products include antiseptics, antibiotics, detergents, surfactants, saline, and water. Wound cleansing will not effectively debride a wound that has substantial necrotic tissue [23].

Chronic nonhealing wounds can endanger patients' well being. Bone infection (osteomyelitis), septicemia, and generalized sepsis seriously threaten patients' lives. Even without progressing to this level of severity, large chronically nonhealing wounds can lose large amounts of protein [24].

Optimal wound debridement is based on comprehensive patient and wound assessment. For example, a necrotic pressure ulcer will not improve despite quality debridement processes if the true causative factor (pressure) is not reduced or eliminated. Experienced clinicians can attest to the fact that previously treated pressure ulcers may develop new necrotic tissue if further pressure damage ensues. Similarly, no degree of debridement will control the venous hypertension associated with venous stasis ulcers. Once basic causes are addressed effectively, debridement of the wound bed can progress. Mounting evidence supports good wound cleansing, and debridement enhances wound healing. If gentle nontoxic cleansing does not remove superficial necrotic, nonviable tissue then other debridement methods should be enacted [25].

One caveat is noteworthy. Successful wound debridement will make a wound look bigger (and possibly worse) to nonprofessionals. The enlargement of the wound is actually promoting healing. Documentation by the wound care professional should alert clinicians and appropriate significant others that debridement will likely make a wound look as if it is deteriorating before it will eventually improve.

What does nonviable tissue look like? Necrotic tissue generally takes two forms: slough and eschar. Slough is dead tissue that is moist and stringy and yellow, tan, gray, or greenish-gray in color. Eschar is desiccated dead tissue that looks leathery and may vary from thick to thin. Eschar is most often black but can also be red or tannish brown. Both slough and eschar are attached to the wound bed [4,26,27].

A critically important concept grounds the optimal use of debridement. Some wounds should not be debrided. An extremity ulcer with stable eschar is an example. For a limb without good blood supply, the eschar acts as a physiologic barrier to infection. The eschar should not be removed but rather protected. Likewise, a person who is at an end of life stage and has poor peripheral perfusion should likely not be subjected to invasive surgery. Not all patients with necrotic wounds need surgery before they die. Conversely, it is also central to optimal care to recognize when debridement is needed urgently. A person who has diabetes mellitus and presents with a necrotic foot ulcer that has clinical signs of infection (induration, fever, erythema, and exudate) needs surgical debridement in the immediate future [28].

Evidence-based practice and wound debridement

Traditionally, wound care and wound debridement specifically have been grounded in best practices approaches. Best practice approaches have been based on expert opinion, tradition, and anecdotal experience. In contemporary health care, best practice approaches are acceptable in areas where there is insufficient evidence to generate evidence-based guidelines [29].

More recently, wound debridement approaches have been scrutinized, and a more rigorous evidence base is emerging. The need to remove necrotic tissue is widely accepted. Indeed, the National Guideline Clearinghouse [30], in its recommendations for pressure ulcer treatment, stated that necrotic tissues should be debrided based on patient condition, treatment goals, and the amount of necrotic tissue in the wound bed. They gave this statement a "D4" rating, that is, the recommendation is based on existing high quality evidence-based guidelines. However, no randomized controlled trials have been conducted that examine the effect of healing of debridement versus no debridement of chronic wounds [4]. Indeed, to generate such a trial would create substantial ethical dilemmas for its researchers.

Evidence for the effectiveness of different methods of debridement is generally lacking, and methods of measurement are poorly controlled [8]. Fortunately, some controlled trials are beginning to elucidate the "best" methods in selected situations and in comparison with other methods. For example, Sherman [31] studied a cohort of 103 patients with 145 ulcers. Sixty-one of 70 patients received maggot or conventional treatment of wounds (moisture retentive dressings). He found that maggot debridement therapy was statistically significantly better in achieving greater and faster debridement than conventional therapy.

A recent Cochrane Library Review [32] examined five randomized controlled trials of debridement of diabetic foot ulcers. Three trials used hydrogel compared with two trials that used sharp debridement and one trial that used larval therapy. The pooled analysis showed that the hydrogels were significantly more effective than gauze or standard care in healing diabetic foot ulcers. Reviews such as this are extremely limited, to date. Another recent study [33] examined the efficacy of two enzymatic agents (collagenase and papain-urea) on pressure ulcer debridement. The researchers concluded that debridement was more rapid with the papain-urea formulation. In 1999, Bradley et al [34] reviewed 35 randomized controlled trials and summarized the evidence for relative effectiveness of different debridement methods. The studies used dextranomer beads, cadexomer iodine, hydrogels, enzymatic agents, zinc oxide tape, surgery, or sharp debridement, and maggots. The authors concluded that evidence was insufficient to promote one debridement method over another. Steed et al [35] found in a retrospective review of data on diabetics with plantar ulcers with good blood supply that frequent sharp debridement coupled with recombinant growth factor therapy had a higher rate of healing versus those patients who underwent growth factor therapy alone.

Despite recent endeavors, generally, knowledge about the optimal frequency, extent, and type of debridement is limited [19]. Systematic literature reviews of controlled clinical trials will become increasingly available from multiple sources such as the Cochrane Library and the American College of Physicians Journal Club. For the greatest level of support, systematic reviews should include only true experimental studies [29].

One way in which these systematic reviews are linked to patient care is clinical practice guidelines. These guidelines include available research evidence such as reviews of controlled clinical trials plus other available evidence pertaining to treatment and evaluation of outcomes. These guidelines are generally broader in scope. Clinical practice guidelines for wound care are available from many sources such as the Wound, Ostomy, Continence Nurses Society (www.wocn.org), the National Guideline Clearinghouse (www.guideline.gov), and the Agency for Healthcare Research and Quality (www.ahrq.gov/clinic/epcix.htm), to name only a few [36]. Wound debridement approaches will likely become more streamlined as available systematic reviews and clinical practice guidelines guide information-seeking clinicians.

No systematic review can replace critical clinical expertise. Once clinicians determine that wound bed debridement is necessary and safe, they need to select an appropriate method or methods, cognizant of how debridement processes work and the advantages and disadvantages associated with them. In this way, correct methods can be listed to appropriate patients. A recent consensus project [5] enacted by national wound care specialists developed an algorithm to assist clinicians to choose the method of debridement matching either primary, secondary, or maintenance debridement needs.

Methods of wound debridement

Multiple methods are available for wound debridement, including surgical or sharp, mechanical, chemical, autolytic, enzymatic, biotherapeutic, laser, and "other" methods. Some methods are considered "selective" in that they remove only the necrotic or devitalized tissue. Nonselective methods remove normal as well as necrotic tissue. For obvious reasons, selective methods are usually preferred. Generally, there is no one best approach. Each method is appropriate for certain clinical situations and may be used in combination effectively—and so goes the search for the ultimate debridement tool or method. Rather, the choice of debridement method depends on multiple contextual factors associated with the patient and the wound (Box 1). To assist with debridement method choice, various algorithms are becoming available that focus on chronic wound care [7]. However, optimal use of wound bed debridement techniques ultimately depends on education and experience. Table 1 contains the various methods of debridement with advantages and disadvantages associated with each. An interesting phenomenon is occurring related to wound debridement methods. Older more "alternative" methods are reemerging as legitimate methods of topical therapy and debridement. These methods include biotherapy (eg, maggots) and the use of natural substances that can be categorized as "other" types of debridement, including the topical use of honey. In three recent controlled clinical trials [37], honey was associated with faster healing in superficial burns than transparent dressings or silver sulfadiazine. Honey is also associated with autolytic debridement, deodorizing action, and an antibacterial action.

Patient and family wishes must be considered along with best available evidence. Sometimes a best practices approach is not taken because a patient does not wish aggressive (or conversely, conservative) therapy.

Quality patient education and cultural competence and sensitivity play critical roles in the use of debridement approaches. In today's multicultural

---

Box 1. Factors influencing choice of wound debridement method

Amount of debris
Available time for debridement
Cost of debridement process
Nature of care setting
Patient allergies
Patient's pain level
Patient's prognosis and treatment plan
Patient's wishes and opinions
Potential patient problems
Maceration of wound
Tissue trauma
Bleeding (hemorrhage)
Presence of infection
Size of wound
Skill of the clinician
Type of debris
Type of exudate
Wound depth and undermining and tunneling

Table 1
Types and methods of debridement

Method/Definition	Advantages	Disadvantages	Contraindications
Surgical/Conservative Sharp Selective Use of instruments to remove necrotic tissue from wound bed. The instruments can include scalpel, forceps, and scissors	Fast and effective Selective to only necrotic tissue May be performed by specially educated nurses, therapists, and physicians Can be performed at bedside for smaller wounds Preferred method when debridement is urgently indicated (eg, sepsis)	Analgesia/anesthesia required especially for bedside usage Substantial costs included Painful Requires discernment of viable vs nonviable tissue Potential for bacteremia and sequelae Need to assess for blood dyscrasias and anticoagulant effects Requires special training and/or licensure Extensive surgical debridement requires patient's written consent Large size wounds usually require an operating room visit	Bleeding disorders Patient instability or severe immune compromise Ischemic extremity Lack of expertise in procedure Densely adherent tissue in which interface between viable and necrotic tissue is not clear With great caution in anti-coagulated patient [7,8,40–42]
Mechanical Nonselective Wet-to-dry dressings Moist saline sponge placed in wound is allowed to dry; removal of dry gauze removes devitalized tissue	Good for larger wounds with substantial devitalized assue Good for nonsurgical candidates	Painful Not cost effective; requires several daily dressing changes Non selective; removes both healthy and necrotic tissue Gauze fibers can embed in wound creating foreign body reaction Potential for maceration of surrounding skin Trauma to capillaries may cause bleeding	Clean granulating wound [4,7,24,26,38,41,42,49,51]

Hydrotherapy Also called whirlpool; Places patient in bath in which warmed swirling water softens and removes devitalized tissue	Excellent for cleansing wound and surrounding tissue Usually provides a degree of increased comfort for patient Increases circulation to wound surface	May disperse bacteria on removal Does not provide thermal protection or bacterial barrier Dated method given other modern therapies available Requires patient transport May overtraumatize wound bed May macerate peri-wound skin May increase risk for waterborne infections such as *Pseudomonas aeruginosa* Requires disinfection of whirlpool tank Requires care worker protection from aerosolization via personal protective equipment Can increase venous congestion in lower extremities exacerbating venous hypertension	Clean granulating wounds Diabetics with severe neuropathy [24,26,47]
Pulsed lavage Use of specialized equipment that allows pulsating irrigation with fluid (often saline) with combined suction	Permits variation of pulsed fluid pressures (ideally 4–15 psi) Excellent for bed-bound patients	May be painful; may require premedication May drive harmful organisms deeper into tissue	Clean granulating wound [24,40]
Chemical Nonselective Hypochlorites (eg, Dakin's solution)	Helps debride necrotic slowly Lowers microbial count	Deleterious to healing tissue and wound healing cells Possible irritant effects on surrounding peri-wound skin	Clean, noninfected wounds [4,42,54]

(continued on next page)

Table 1 (*continued*)

Method/Definition	Advantages	Disadvantages	Contraindications
Hydrogen peroxide	Desloughing agent Has some bactericidal effect	Deleterious to healing tissue and wound healing cells Possible irritant effects on surrounding peri-wound skin Theoretical risk of air embolism	Clean granulating wound [4]
Povidone iodine	Cheap and readily available Broad spectrum of antimicrobial activity May help dry slough for easier sharp debridement	Deleterious to fibroblasts in therapeutic dilutions Stains tissue	Clean, noninfected wound Iodine allergy [4,7,46]
Cadexomer iodine (eg, Iodosorb, Iodoflex)	Slow-release Safe for cellular viability and absorbs exudates Can absorb up to 7 times its weight Comes as ointment or dressing Helps with autolytic debridement Stimulates wound healing process	Safe for fibroblasts and other wound healing cells Used with caution in patients with thyroid disease	Clean, noninfected wound [4,26,46]
Autolytic Selective Use of body's own wound fluid enzymes to liquefy necrotic tissue; accomplished through moisture-retentive topical therapy. Some types fully occlude whereas others are semi-occlusive Hydrocolloids, act to retain body's own moisture in wound	Safe and slowly effective Patient comfort, usually soothing by covering open nerve endings Associated with decreased risk of wound infection Indicated when no urgent clinical need for drainage or removal of revitalized tissue Good choice for patients who are not surgical candidates Easy to perform Performed in any care setting	Works slowly compared with other methods Cannot be used in certain situations (eg, occlusive dressing over eschar in pulseless extremity or infected wound) Requires constant monitoring of wound for infection in immune-compromised patients Must assess blood supply in extremity Hydrocolloid dressing fluid odor often mistaken for "infected"	Infected ulcers or wounds Cellulitic wounds Deep extensive wound Severe neutropenia With great caution in immune compromised and frail elderly [4,7,24,26,30,41,42,52]

Hydrogels, donate water into necrotic tissue to liquefy it Alginates Foam Hydrofiber Moisture vapor permeable, transparent, film, retains body's own moisture in wound	Hydrogels, alginates, foams and hydrofibers will absorb some wound fluid Maintain moist wound therapy All except for moisture vapor permeable dressings can be used in deep extensive wounds to good effect	Absorptive dressings can dry out wound bed if not discontinued when appropriate	Dry wound bed not appropriate for absorptive dressings [4,7,24,26,30,41,42,52]
Enzymatic Selective Protein agents (enzymes) that work by degrading and debriding necrotic tissue by digesting and dissolving it Types available include: Collagenase (Santyl) Papain-urea (Accuzyme) Papain-urea and chlorophyllin (Panafil)	Safe for patient use if used according to directions Good for settings with no sharp debridement available Good for patients receiving anticoagulants Good for patients who have contraindications to surgery Decrease wound trauma Good for home care patient Cost effective if used properly Selectively removes necrotic tissue Will not harm normal tissue Sometimes used with topical antibiotics (not always evidence-based) Can be used in infected wounds	Usually not effective for advanced cellulitic wounds Require physician or prescriber's order Slower and less aggressive than sharp debridement Cannot be used with other common wound products such as metal ions (eg, Silvadene) or with topical antiseptics (eg, Dakin's solution) Some agents require or recommend cross-hatching of eschar with a scalpel Expensive Sometimes associated with peri-wound inflammation Temporary burning sensation Knowing when to stop therapy Papain-urea has been associated rarely with anaphylaxis	Clean granulating wound Allergies Use papain-urea type agent with great caution in latex allergy patient [1,4,7,19,24,41,43,45,48]

(continued on next page)

Table 1 (*continued*)

Method/Definition	Advantages	Disadvantages	Contraindications
Biotherapy Selective Also called maggot debridement therapy or biosurgery Use of sterile maggots for debriding wounds Uses larvae of *Lucilia sericata* (greenbottle fly); maggots secrete proteolytic enzymes that break down tissue	Removes only necrotic tissue Relatively inexpensive Painless Acts relatively rapidly Can be used on all ages of patients Can be used on immobilized persons and pregnant women Can be used concurrently with antibiotics Has multiple indications including: pressure ulcers, vascular ulcers, diabetic ulcers, traumatic and post surgical wounds, burns, and methicillin-resistant *S. aureus*-infected wounds	Some patients find too offensive to accept, "yuck factor" Potential for allergic reaction Cannot use in tunneling wounds Ineffective for osteomyelitis Secretions irritate healthy skin Increased pain with use in ischemic wounds Dressing change is time consuming	Patient with allergies to eggs, soybeans, and fly larvae Lack of wound hemostasis Adhesive allergies Deep tracked wounds [41,43,44,45,46,55,56]
Wound VAC (hypobaric therapy) Selective A sub-atmospheric pressure dressing that creates a closed wound system-applies 125 mm Hg of pressure	Removes interstitial fluid/edema Assists with granulation Acts to liquefy and remove slough and soften eschar Decreases bacterial count Can grow granulation tissue over bone and tendon	Can be painful Expensive Can cause pressure necrosis if not applied skillfully Requires electrical supply	Hemorrhage Exposed blood vessels High output enteric fistula [40,47]

Laser Selective	Debrides only necrotic tissue Decreases edema by sealing lymphatics May stimulate wound healing	Requires special equipment Requires patient and user protective gear	Clean granulating wound [17,25]
Other Selective Topical Substances Honey Use of medicinal honey usually applied by special dressings	Debrides necrotic tissues through osmotic effect of sugar Has broad spectrum antibacterial like effect Has deodorizing anti-inflammatory and anti-scarring effects Used on variety of wound including: burns, surgical wounds, necrotizing fasciitis, and chronic ulcers Cheap Not painful Can be used across care settings	May require operating room visit Slower debridement Rare adverse allergic reactions Transient stinging sensation	None reported [37,50,53]

Data from references [1,4,7,8,17,19,24,26,30,37,38,40–56].

society, caregivers must be cognizant of ethnic and religious preferences. In the author's experience, patients or caregivers may be uncooperative with debridement approaches based on erroneous interpretations or perceptions. For example, a patient and his family initially refused an enzymatic debriding process because they thought it contained substances proscribed by their religion. Another patient feared a negative pressure wound device because it would injure (electrically shock) him. Both patients agreed to therapy when full processes and ingredients were explained and documentation was shared.

Another component of patient education regarding debridement is the need for ongoing debridement in chronic wounds [20]. Maintenance debridement is necessary in chronic wounds in which the underlying pathology is associated with continuous recurrence of slough and eschar. Patients need to be counseled that continuing debridement does not constitute treatment failure or poor patient compliance.

Although the armamentarium of wound debridement methods has expended substantially, recent research [38] has substantiated that the most traditional, cost ineffective method, saline wet to dry gauze, persists in being the most commonly used approach even in circumstances for which there is little evidence to support its use (clean open surgical wounds healing by secondary intention). These researchers and other authors suggest that tradition, lack of education, and poor understanding of cost efficacy drive many physicians' debridement choices [39].

Summary

Wound debridement is a critical component of promoting optimal healing for a wound with necrotic tissue. Although much is known about the multiple barriers to healing that necrotic detritus presents, much is still unknown about the best ways, timing, and approaches to constructing a healthy wound bed. Falanga's [2] "black box," a metaphor for the unknown components of wound healing and debridement, should remind all practitioners that future research needs to address the continuing questions and issues associated with promotion of quality chronic wound healing outcomes.

Suggested reading

Armstrong DG, Lavery LA, Masquez JR, et al. How and why to surgically debride neuropathic diabetic foot wounds. JAPMA 2002;92(7):402–4.

Ashworth J. Conservative sharp debridement: the professional and legal issues. Prof Nurse 2002; 17(10):585–8.

Brown GS. Reporting outcomes for stage IV pressure ulcer healing: a proposal. Adv Skin Wound Care 2000;13:277–83.

Campton-Johnston S, Wilson J. Infected wound management: advanced technologies, moisture-retentive dressings, and die-hard methods. Crit Care Nurs Q 2001;24(2):64–77.

Capasso VA, Munro BH. The cost and efficacy of two wound treatments. AORN J 2003;77(5): 984–1004.

Copson D. Evaluating a new technique for the treatment of chronic wounds. Prof Nurse 2000; 17(12):729–33.

Dharmarajan TS, Ahmed S. The growing problems of pressure ulcers. Postgrad Med 2003;113(5): 77–85.

Falabella A. Debridement of wounds. Wounds 1998;10:1C–9C.

Fink A, Deluca G. Necrotizing fasciitis: pathophysiology and treatment. Medsurg Nurs 2003; 11(1):33–6.

Hahn JF, Olsen CL, Tomaselli N, et al. Wounds: nursing care and product selection: part II. Nursing Spectrum Career Fitness Online 2002; www.nursingspectrum.com/ce/ce81.html. Accessed December 27, 2003.

Harding K, Cutting K, Price P. The cost effectiveness of wound management protocols of care. Br J Nurs 2000;9(19):S4–24.

Hawkins-Bradley B, Walden M. Treatment of a non-healing wound with hypergranulation tissue and rolled edges. J Wound Ostomy Continence Nurs 2002;29(6):320–4.

Holloway S, Ryder J. Management of a patient with postoperative necrotizing fasciitis. Br J Nurs 2002;11(16):525–32.

Morison MJ. A framework for patient assessment and care planning. In: Morison MJ, Ovington L, Wilkie K, editors. Chronic wound care: a problem based learning approach. Edinburgh: CV Mosby; 2004. p. 46–66.

Wound Ostomy Continence Nurses Society. Position statement: conservative sharp wound debridement for registered nurses 1996. http://www.wocn.org/publications/posstate/debride. html. Accessed December 27, 2003.

References

[1] Falanga V. Wound bed preparation and the role of enzymes: a case for multiple action of therapeutic agents. Wounds 2002;14(2):47–57.

[2] Falanga V. Wound bed preparation: future approaches. Ostomy Wound Manage 2003; 49(5A)(Suppl):S30–3.

[3] Kirsner R. Wound bed preparation. Ostomy Wound Manage 2003;49(5A)(Suppl):S2–3.

[4] O'Brien M. Exploring methods of wound debridement. Br J Community Nurs 2003; 7(Suppl 1):S10–8.

[5] Ayello E, Dowsett C, Schultz G, et al. Time heals all wounds. Nursing 2004;34(4):36–42.

[6] Sibbald RG, Orsted H, Schultz GS, et al. For the international wound bed preparation advisory board and the Canadian chronic wound advisory board. Preparing the wound bed 2003: focus on infection and inflammation. Ostomy Wound Manage 2003;49(11):24–51.

[7] Sibbald RG, Williamson D, Orsted HL, et al. Preparing the wound bed–debridement, bacterial balance, and moisture balance. Ostomy Wound Manage 2000;46(11):14–35.

[8] Leaper D. Sharp technique for wound debridement. World Wide Wounds. Available at: http://www.worldwidewounds.com/2002/december/leaper/sharp-debridement.html. Accessed February 6, 2004.

[9] Robson MC, Stenberg BD, Heggers JP. Wound healing alterations caused by infection. Clin Plast Surg 1990;17:485–92.

[10] Zacur H, Kirsner RS. Debridement: rationale and therapeutic options. Wounds 2002; 14(Suppl 7):S25–65.

[11] Serralta VW, Harrison-Balestra C, Cazzaniga AL, et al. Lifestyles of bacteria in wounds: presence of biofilms? Wounds 2001;13(1):29–34.

[12] Wysocki AB. Evaluating and managing open skin wounds: colonization versus infection. AACN Clin Issues 2002;13(3):382–97.

[13] Kerstein MD, Reis ED. Current surgical perspectives in wound healing. Wounds 2001;13(2): 53–8.

[14] Mulder GD, Vandeberg JS. Cellular senescence and matrix metalloprotease activity in chronic wounds. JAPMA 2002;92(1):34–7.

[15] Hunt TK, Hopf H, Hussain Z. Physiology of wound healing. Adv Skin Wound Care 2000; 13(Suppl 2):S6–11.

[16] Baharestani M. The clinical relevance of debridement. In: Baharestani M, Gottrup F, Holstein P, et al, editors. The clinical relevance of debridement. Berlin: Springer-Verlag; 1999. p. 1–16.

[17] Dolynchuk K. Debridement. In: Krasner DL, Rodeheaver GT, Sibbald RG, editors. Chronic wound care: a clinical sourcebook for healthcare professionals. 3rd edition. Wayne (PA): HMP Communication; 2001. p. 385–90.

[18] Chakrabarty A, Phillips T. Diagnostic dilemmas in pyoderma gangrenosum. Wounds 2002; 14:302–5.

[19] Ennis WJ, Meneses P. Wound healing at the local level: the stunned wound. Ostomy Wound Manage 2000;46(IA):395–485.

[20] Schultz G, Sibbald RG, Falanga V, et al. Wound bed preparation: a systematic approach to wound management. Wound Repair Regen 2003;11:1–20.

[21] Hall P, Schumann L. Wound care: meeting the challenge. J Am Acad Nurse Pract 2001;13(6): 258–68.

[22] Stotts N, Wipke-Tevis D. Co-factors in impaired wound healing. In: Krasner DL, Rodeheaver GT, Sibbald RG, editors. Chronic wound care: a clinical sourcebook for healthcare professionals. Wayne (PA): HMP Communications; 2001. p. 265–72.

[23] Ovington LG, Eisenbud D. Dressings and cleansing agents. In: Morison MJ, Ovington L, Wilkie K, editors. Chronic wound care: a problem-based learning approach. Edinburgh: CV Mosby; 2004. p. 117–28.

[24] Ayello E, Cuddigan J, Kerstein M. Skip the knife: debriding wounds without surgery. Nursing 2002;32(9):58–63.

[25] Dolynchuk K, Keast D, Campbell K, et al. Best practices for the prevention and treatment of pressure ulcers. Ostomy Wound Manage 2000;46(11):38–52.

[26] Nelson D, Dilloway MA. Principles, products, and practical aspects of wound care. Crit Care Nurs Q 2002;25(1):33–54.

[27] Tong A. Recognizing, managing and removing slough. NT Plus 2000;96(29):15–6.

[28] Krasner DL. How to prepare the wound bed. Ostomy Wound Manage 2001;47(4): 59–61.

[29] Gray M, Beitz J, Colwell J, et al. Evidence-based nursing practice II: advanced concepts for WOC nursing practice. J Wound Ostomy Continence Nurs 2004;31(2):53–61.

[30] Singapore Ministry of Health. Nursing management of pressure ulcers in adults. Singapore: Ministry of Health. 2001. http://www.guideline.gov/summary/summary.aspx?doc_id= 3276.html. Accessed January 28, 2004.

[31] Sherman RA. Maggot versus conservative debridement therapy for the treatment of pressure ulcers. Wound Repair Regen 2002;10(4):208.

[32] Smith J. Debridement of diabetic foot ulcers [abstract]. Cochrane Library. Chichester, (UK): Wiley & Sons; 2003. p. 4.

[33] Alvarez OM, Fernandez-Obregon A, Rogers RS, et al. Chemical debridement of pressure ulcers: a prospective, randomized, comparative trial of collagenase and papain/urea formulations. Wounds 2000;12(12):15–25.

[34] Bradley M, Cullum N, Sheldon T. The debridement of chronic wounds: a systematic review. Health Tech Assess 1999;3(17) [executive summary: 1–4].

[35] Steed DL, Donohue D, Webster MW. Effect of extensive debridement and treatment on the healing of diabetic foot ulcers. J Am Coll Surg 1996;183:61–4.

[36] Ryan S, Perrier L, Sibbald RG. Searching for evidence-based medicine in wound care: an introduction. Ostomy Wound Manage 2003;49(11):67–75.

[37] Molan P. Re-introducing honey in the management of wounds and ulcers–theory and practice. Ostomy Wound Manage 2002;48(11):28–40.

[38] Armstrong M, Price P. Wet-to-dry gauze dressings: fact and fiction. Wounds 2004;16(2): 56–62.

[39] Van Rijswijk L, Beitz J. The traditions and terminology of wound dressings: food for thought. J Wound Ostomy Continence Nurs 1998;25(3):116–22.

[40] Attinger CE, Bulan E, Blume PA. Surgical debridement: the key to successful wound healing and reconstruction. Clin Podiatr Med Surg 2000;17(4):599–630.

[41] Ayello E, Baranoski S, Kerstein M, et al. Wound debridement. In: Baranoski S, Ayello E, editors. Wound care essentials: practice principles. Philadelphia: Lippincott, Williams & Wilkins; 2003. p. 117–26.

[42] Burns P. Wound bed preparation: essentials for wound care–debridement, bacterial balance, and exudate management. The Remington Report 2003;May/June:7–9.

[43] Claxton MJ, Armstrong DG, Short B, et al. 5 questions and answers about maggot debridement therapy. Adv Skin Wound Care 2003;16(2):99–102.

[44] Dossey L. Maggots and leeches: when science and aesthetics collide. Altern Ther Health Med 2002;8(4):12–6, 106.

[45] Drisdelle R. Maggot debridement therapy. Nursing 2003;33(6):17.

[46] Drosou A, Falabella A, Kirsner RS. Antiseptics on wounds: an area of controversy. Wounds 2003;15(5):149–66.

[47] Hess CL, Howard MA, Attinger CE. A review of mechanical adjuncts in wound healing: hydrotherapy, ultrasound, negative pressure, therapy, hyperbaric oxygen, and electro-stimulation. Ann Plast Surg 2003;51(2):210–8.

[48] Hewitt H, Wint Y, Talabere L, et al. The use of papaya on pressure ulcers: a natural alternative. Am J Nurs 2002;102(12):73–7.

[49] Lee SK, Turnbull GB. Wound care: What's really cost effective? Nursing Homes Long-Term Care Management 2001;50(4):40–4, 74–5.

[50] World Wide Wounds. Honey as a topical antibacterial agent for treatment of infected wounds. Molan P. http://www.worldwidewounds.com/2001/november/molan/honey-as-topical-agent.html. Accessed February 6, 2004.

[51] Ovington L. Hanging wet to dry dressings out to dry. Adv Skin Wound Care 2002;15(2): 79–84.

[52] Ovington LG. Wound care products: how to choose. Home Healthc Nurse 2001;19(4): 224–32.

[53] Pieper B, Caliri M. Nontraditional wound care: a review of the evidence for the use of sugar, papaya/papain, and fatty acids. J Wound Ostomy Continence Nurs 2003;30:175–83.

[54] Stotts N. Wound infection: diagnosis and management. In: Morison MJ, Ovington L, Wilkie K, editors. Chronic wound care: a problem-based learning approach. Edinburgh: CV Mosby; 2004. p. 101–16.

[55] Thomas S. The use of sterile maggots in wound management. NT Plus 2002;98(36):45–6.

[56] Thomas S, Jones M. Wound debridement: evaluating the costs. Nurs Stand 2001;15(22): 59–61.

NURSING
CLINICS
OF NORTH AMERICA

Nurs Clin N Am 40 (2005) 251–265

Support Surfaces: Beds, Mattresses, Overlays—Oh My!

Dianne Mackey, BSN, RN, PHN, CWOCN

8996 Gainsborough Avenue, San Diego, CA 92129, USA

Inherent in almost all guidelines and protocols that address the prevention and treatment of pressure ulcers is the use of support surfaces. The market is inundated with a wide array of support surfaces, but very little research exists that evaluates their efficacy and effectiveness. The product technologies at times are overlapping and lack clear definition, which further complicates the decision-making ability of the clinician. Confusion and controversy remain, as nurses struggle to recommend a support surface for an individual patient or for an entire facility. The lack of standardization in testing products and reporting outcomes and the development and use of a common language are a few of the challenges that face each of us in our daily practices. The manufacturers of these products are continually striving to fit their products in the Medicare Part B Support Surface Policy [1], which was drafted and implemented in January, 1996. It is imperative that the products covered under this policy represent the most current technology and address the pressure and shear and friction forces that lead to the development of pressure ulcers.

This article presents the current understanding of the scientific evidence relating to the efficacy of support surfaces, along with risk factors that contribute to skin breakdown. The different classes and features of support surfaces and the reimbursement structure across the care continuum are summarized. Finally, an update on the National Pressure Ulcer Advisory Panel's sponsored Support Surface Initiative will be presented.

Background

Pressure ulcers are a major concern for health care workers and for patients with restricted mobility or chronic disease and for the elderly.

E-mail address: diannern@san.rr.com

Researchers have found that pressure ulcers are a significant, independent predictor of both hospital costs and lengths of stay. Several studies have shown that patients who develop pressure ulcers that are stage II or higher have lengths of stay that range from 4 to 8 days longer, with costs ranging from $1,877 to $15,229 more than patients without pressure ulcers [2]. The Centers for Disease Control Injury Research Agenda [3] reports that an estimated 200,000 people in the United States live with spinal cord injuries and that this number increases annually by as many as 11,000 individuals. Pressure ulcers, a secondary condition of spinal cord injuries, are a common cause of lost productivity. Studies [4–6] demonstrate that 3% to 10% of the population in both hospital and community health care settings acquire some degree of pressure damage. In 1990, the incidence for pressure ulcer development in nursing homes was 13.2%. According to data from the Minimum Data Set, between 1991 and 1996, the risk-adjusted rate of new pressure ulcers has been reported to decrease by 25%; between the years 1977 and 1987, the increased liability associated with this adverse outcome had a median settlement of $250,000 [7].

According to Aronovitch [11], approximately 1.6 million patients develop hospital-acquired pressure ulcers, at a cost of $2.2 to $3.6 billion per year. Of the ulcers acquired in this population, 23% occur in surgical patients undergoing procedures lasting more than 3 hours and represent an annual direct cost of $750 million to $1.5 billion. This cost is estimated to be 2.5 times the cost of prevention [2].

Defining the evidence

The Blue Cross/Blue Shield Technical Evaluation Center report of 1998 attempted to answer questions relating to the effectiveness of support surfaces. According to Conine [8], effectiveness is defined by answering the question "What are the practical characteristics or the impact of a new maneuver when introduced into practice?" or "How usable is the product in practical, everyday real conditions?" In defining efficacy, the author states that efficacy answers the question "To what degree does the treatment work or result in the intended outcomes under carefully controlled unbiased conditions [eg, randomized controlled clinical trial]" [8]. By looking at evidence of randomized controlled clinical trials only, the Technical Evaluation Center report conclusions may answer questions about efficacy but not effectiveness. These conclusions address the types of support surfaces as outlined in the 1996 Medicare Part B Support Surface Policy [1]. The conclusions are 1) compared with patients placed on control surfaces, patients placed on Group I and Group II surfaces were less likely to develop pressure ulcers; and 2) compared with Group I surfaces, treatment with Group II surfaces improved health outcomes (healing) of patients with pressure ulcers.

These conclusions do not come as a surprise, considering the limitations and narrow scope of the randomized controlled clinical trials. What is overlooked is the importance of clinical expertise and consensus when the scientific literature is incomplete or inconsistent [9].

The 2001 Cochrane Database of Systematic Reviews [10] of support surfaces reports that after searching 19 databases, including a hand search of journals, conference proceedings, and bibliographies, only 37 eligible randomized, controlled trials were found. Twenty-nine trials involved patients without preexisting pressure ulcers; six trials involved patients with pressure ulcers; and two trials evaluated support surface effects for both prevention and treatment. Three of the studies evaluated different operating table surfaces.

The results of the Cochrane database of support surfaces

Prevention

Twenty-nine randomized controlled trials through 2000 showed that some high end foam mattresses were more effective than "standard" hospital mattresses for moderate- to high-risk patients. Additionally, limited evidence suggests that low air loss beds reduce the incidence of pressure ulcers in intensive care. Three operating room trials [11,12,13] indicated that pressure-reducing overlays (air and gel) used on the operating table may be beneficial in reducing the subsequent incidence of pressure ulcers in high-risk surgical patients.

Treatment

There is good evidence that air-fluidized and low air loss beds improve healing rates. The relative merits of alternating air and constant low pressure surfaces are unclear. In summary, based on the most current scientific evidence, it is impossible to determine the most effective surface for either prevention or treatment [10].

The working "evidence" points to the fact that there is no doubt that patients at high risk or those with pressure damage need an improved support surface. To state that "it works" is no longer good enough. Consistent and appropriate selection of support surfaces is necessary to promote positive clinical outcomes while maintaining patient comfort and controlling costs. Our individual protocols and guidelines enshrine this fact.

In 1992 and 1994, the Agency for Health care Policy and Research (now called the Agency for Healthcare Research and Quality) [14,15] developed clinical practice guidelines that address both the prevention and treatment of pressure ulcers. In 2003, the Wound Ostomy & Continence Nurses Society (WOCN) published a guide titled "Guideline for Prevention and Management of Pressure Ulcers" [16]. These documents address the important role that support surfaces play in the prevention and treatment of pressure ulcers.

Risk factors

In discussing support surface selection, it is important to acknowledge the extrinsic and intrinsic factors that lead to the development of skin breakdown. According to Bergstrom et al [15], factors that contribute to pressure ulcer development affect the pressure over a bony prominence and the tolerance of the tissues to pressure. There is an inverse relationship between time and pressure; neither time nor pressure alone causes tissue ischemia, however, pressure multiplied by duration of time can create an ulcer [17].

Mobility, sensory loss, and activity level are related to the concept of increasing pressure. Extrinsic factors (shear, friction, and moisture) and intrinsic factors (nutrition, age, and arteriolar pressure) relate to the concept of tissue tolerance. Emotional stress, temperature, smoking, and interstitial fluid flow may influence pressure ulcer development. These lesions profoundly affect the quality of life for patients and their caregivers and are often associated with serious infections, pain, and even death.

Support surface requirements

The general consensus among clinicians who are faced with the difficult decision concerning which support surface to choose is that the surface needs to address four areas of performance: pressure redistribution, including immersion and envelopment, shear and friction management, temperature, and moisture control. Pressure redistribution is a term that replaces the terms pressure reduction and pressure relief, because there has never been consensus about how to measure and define these two terms. Pressure redistribution is the function or ability of a support surface to distribute load over the surface or contact area [18]. It is the ability of the support surface to equalize the loading on the body or distribute loading away from bony prominences or other at-risk sites. Immersion and envelopment are two concepts associated with pressure redistribution. Immersion refers to the linear depth into which a body submerges in a support surface [18]. The more immersed a patient is, the greater the surface area of contact; and, given a constant body weight, the more surface area, the lower the overall pressure (pressure = force ÷ area). Immersion comes at a cost, however, because a body can sink too far into a soft surface resulting in the patient lying on a hard surface, so just being soft is not enough. Envelopment is the capability of a support surface to conform to or encompass the contours of the human body [18]. An enveloping surface should have the ability to conform to irregularities in contours of body shape, objects in pockets, clothing, and other forms, without causing a substantial increase in pressure.

An ideal enveloping surface (such as a fluid without a container) would maximize contact area and eliminate areas of high loading over bony prominences or other at-risk sites. Presently no perfect enveloping support surfaces exist, but the goal is to find those surfaces that perform better than others [18].

Currently, there are no widely accepted clinical methods for measuring the viability of tissue over a bony prominence when it is subjected to the distress of prolonged pressure. The most reliable and easily obtained measurement is tissue interface pressure. Tissue interface pressure is the force per unit area that acts perpendicularly between the body and the support surface [19]. Various manufacturers have developed pressure mapping devices to quantify an outcome measurement that is believed to provide an approximation of the amount of pressure on a particular bony prominence. Most support surface studies have relied solely on interface pressure measurements. However, with individual variability, interface pressure alone is insufficient to evaluate the efficacy of a particular device or class of devices [17].

Shear is the parallel force that causes internal tissue layers to slide and pull against each other. The disassociation between the connective tissue and blood vessels results in the restriction or interruption of blood and lymph flow into the local muscles and subcutaneous tissue. The most common circumstance for shear occurs when a patient is in the semi-Fowler's position, and the head of the bed is raised, resulting in the patient's skeleton sliding toward the foot of the bed with the skin staying in place (with the help of friction against the bed linen). Shear is the reason many pressure ulcers are much larger than the bony prominence over which they occur. In clinical practice, this partly explains pressure ulcers with large undermined areas [17,20].

Friction occurs when two surfaces move across one another. Friction acts on the epidermal and upper layers of the dermis, leading to an increased susceptibility to a pressure injury. In conjunction with pressure, friction produces ulcerations at lower pressures than pressure alone. In clinical practice, friction can occur when a patient is repositioned or the sheet is adjusted under the patient [17,21].

Moisture and temperature control are variables that have been associated with an increased incidence in pressure ulcer development. Moisture alters the resiliency of the epidermis to external forces. Excess moisture may be caused by urinary or fecal incontinence, perspiration, or wound drainage. Overhydration of the skin also increases the coefficient of friction that contributes to adhesion of the skin to the support surface. This adherence of the weakened skin structures add to shear effects and can promote abrasion, sloughing, and ulceration as the patient moves across the bed surface. The added detrimental effect of fecal incontinence is the presence of bacteria, which can contribute to infection as well as breakdown. Fecal incontinence is highly correlated with pressure ulcer development [21]. Control of temperature at the interface surface (patient-bed boundary) is critical in reducing skin temperature, which in turn slows metabolic activity, decreases circulatory demand, inhibits sweating, and lowers skin hydration. Unfortunately, there are no reported clinical trials that define the optimum level of temperature and moisture reduction by an air loss support system [22].

Support surface characteristics

Effective communication about the various types of support surfaces and the many performance features that each of them offers can be a challenge. It is difficult to get consensus from researchers, clinicians, manufacturers, and engineers on the "language" to use when describing or ordering a pressure redistribution bed, mattress, or overlay. Standardization has become the buzz word in health care as we all strive to speak the same language while incorporating practices that are evidence-based into our daily clinical practices. In an effort to begin communicating effectively, it is helpful to use language that has some universality and agreement among clinicians about which mattress or overlay is the most appropriate, whether it is for an individual patient or for an entire facility. To that end, it is helpful to divide the product line into three categories: technologies, construction, and configuration. Table 1 provides a way to organize this often confusing information and provides a common language when ordering and sharing information about a particular surface.

Support surface selection

Selection of a support surface for an individual or and entire facility can pose many challenges for the novice and the seasoned clinician. It is important to identify and select a support surface with performance characteristics that support the patient goal of prevention or treatment. If prevention is the goal, it is helpful to use the coverage criteria in the 1996

Table 1
Support surfaces characteristics

Support surface technology	Support surface construction	Support surface configuration
Nonpowered (without electricity)	Foam (elastic and viscoelastic)	Overlays
Powered (with electricity)	Fluid-filled (air, water, gel)	Mattress replacement
Low air loss	Hybrid (air/foam, foam/gel)	Full bed systems
Air-fluidized		Bariatric
Hybrid systems (low air loss/ air-fluidized)		

Data from Fleck C. Support surfaces for the 21st century. The Roho Group, April, 2003.

Medicare Part B Support Surface Policy [1]. In that policy, Group I products focus primarily on preventing skin damage and include non-powered overlays and mattresses replacement systems made of foam, air, gel, or water. Powered alternating air overlays with pumps are also included. The following criteria may be used to guide the clinician in choosing the most appropriate and cost-effective surface. Patients are appropriate for a prevention surface if they

1. Are identified as being at-risk for skin breakdown
2. Are able to be repositioned off the ulcer(s)
3. Have more than one turning surface to be turned and repositioned
4. Are placed on products with performance characteristics that prevent or treat partial thickness ulcers
5. Are placed on products that may be used for chronic disease management or pain control, eg, end-stage cancer

These criteria address both patient and product characteristics that assist in the decision-making process about which support surface is appropriate for the prevention of skin breakdown. Although we know that there is insufficient evidence to support the choice of one pressure reduction surface over another for the prevention of pressure ulcers, the WOCN "Guideline for Prevention and Management of Pressure Ulcers" [16] confirms that at-risk patients should not be placed on an ordinary, standard hospital foam mattress. The guideline recommends that at-risk individuals be placed on pressure-reducing surfaces.

If skin breakdown has already occurred and treatment is the goal, the Groups II and III surfaces are the appropriate and cost-effective choices for a support surface. These categories include nonpowered, adjustable zone air or gel overlay and mattress replacement systems, low air loss or alternating air mattress replacement systems and air-fluidized beds. The following criteria may assist the clinician in the selection of a support surface that matches the patient's clinical condition with the most appropriate treatment surface:

1. Products that support the treatment of full thickness pressure ulcers as well as myocutaneous flaps and grafts;
2. Products that address the need for moisture and heat dissipation as well as disease and pain management;
3. Products that are effective in redistributing pressure when the patient presents with pressure ulcers on two or more turning surfaces.

As stated in the WOCN "Guideline for Prevention and Management of Pressure Ulcers" [16] individuals with stage III or IV pressure ulcers or those who have multiple ulcers over several turning surfaces need a pressure-relieving product. Additionally, air fluidized support and low air loss beds are reported as effective treatments and may improve pressure ulcer healing rates. Other selection criteria for support surfaces in general may include

1. Patient's comfort and ability to move independently. The hardness or softness of the surface along with the temperature at the patient-bed boundary may negatively affect the patient's ability to tolerate the surface.
2. Care setting where patient is being provided care. Is there an available and willing family member or caregiver who is able to turn the patient at appropriate intervals? Sometimes the patient is unwilling to cooperate with a turning and repositioning schedule, which in turn puts the patient at an increased risk for skin breakdown.
3. The manufacturer's product warranty and life span, service history, and cost (rental versus purchase). What is the service and maintenance backup availability? A 24-hour call service with on-site repair or replacement is essential. In the home, it is important to know the electrical costs to run products that have a motor or blower and whether there are safety features (ie, visual and audio alarm systems) in case of a power failure.
4. Patient's body weight and build. Most products have a maximum weight for both the actual support surface as well as the bed frame on which it rests. An obese patient may require a surface that will support his or her weight [23–25].

After a product or a range of products is selected for an individual patient or a facility, a continuous process of assessment and reassessment at regular intervals is necessary. As a patient's condition improves, a less aggressive surface may be warranted. Conversely, if a patient's condition begins to deteriorate, the patient may require a higher level of pressure reduction, which may include special features that address shear, friction and moisture [24].

Coverage and reimbursement

As the support surface market continues to grow and the current reimbursement environment continues to shrink, health care professionals need to select therapeutic surfaces with sound information about the effectiveness and efficacy of the products [26]. The WOCN Society developed and published a Fact Sheet (Fig. 1) about support surfaces that clarifies the 1996 Medicare Part B Support Surface policy (coverage criteria, product codes, definitions, and reimbursement in the home setting). Although this national policy covers only home healthcare, many acute care and long-term care facilities that lack decision trees or algorithms have adopted these guidelines to assist the clinician in choosing the most appropriate pressure redistribution surface for their patient population. Although Fig. 1 addresses only the home care setting, Table 2 illustrates coverage and reimbursement for support surfaces in the acute care, long-term care, and hospice settings.

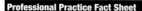

| **Professional Practice Fact Sheet** | | **MEDICARE PART B COVERAGE FOR**
SUPPORT SURFACES IN THE HOME HEALTH SETTING |

Introduction

This fact sheet addresses Medicare Part B support surface coverage criteria and reimbursement guidelines. **These guidelines apply to patients who are eligible for home health care services, but do not apply to acute, longterm or hospice care.**

Coverage Criteria

Group I	Group II	Group III
A patient would qualify if they meet either of the following scenarios:	A patient would qualify if they meet one of the following scenarios:	A patient would qualify only if all of the following criteria are met:
Scenario 1: The patient is completely immobile.	**Scenario 1:** The patient has multiple Stage II ulcers located on the trunk and/or pelvis, and - a comprehensive ulcer treatment program, including the use of an appropriate Group I support surface, has been tried for at least one month. - the ulcers have worsened or remained the same.	- The patient has a Stage III or IV ulcer. - The patient is bedridden or chair bound as a result of severely limited mobility. - In the absence of an air-fluidized bed, the patient would require institutionalization. - The air-fluidized bed is ordered in writing by the patient's attending physician based upon a comprehensive assessment and evaluation.
Scenario 2: The patient has limited mobility or any stage ulcer on the trunk or pelvis and has at least one of the following: - impaired nutritional status - fecal or urinary incontinence - altered sensory perception - compromised circulatory status.	**Scenario 2:** The patient has: - large or multiple Stage III or IV ulcer(s) located on the trunk or pelvis.	- A comprehensive ulcer treatment program, including the use of an appropriate Group II support surface, has been tried for at least one month with worsening or no improvement to the ulcer. - A trained adult caregiver is available to assist the patient with activities of daily living, repositioning, dietary and fluid needs, prescribed treatments, and management and support of the air-fluidized bed system and its problems. - A physician directs the home treatment regimen on a monthly basis. - All other alternative equipment has been considered and ruled out.
	Scenario 3: - The patient has had a recent myocutaneous flap or skin graft on the trunk or pelvis (surgery within the past 60 days). - The patient has been on a Group II or III product prior to discharge from a hospital or skilled nursing facility. Note: Patient coverage under this scenario is limited to 60 days post-op.	An air-fluidized bed will be denied under any of the following circumstances: - Co-existing pulmonary disease - Wet soaks or moist dressings that are not protected with an impervious covering. - Caregiver is unwilling or unable to provide the type of care required on an air-fluidized bed. - Structure support is inadequate to support the weight of the air-fluidized bed. - The electrical system is insufficient for the anticipated increase in consumption.

Wound, Ostomy and Continence Nurses Society ◆ 4700 W. Lake Avenue ◆ Glenview, IL 60025 ◆ www.wocn.org

(page 1 of 4)

Fig. 1. Professional practice fact sheet covering Medicare Part B support surface coverage criteria and reimbursement guidelines. (*From* Wound Ostomy Continence Nurses Society. 4700 W. Lake Ave., Glenview, IL 60025; with permission.)

Professional Practice Fact Sheet	MEDICARE PART B COVERAGE FOR SUPPORT SURFACES IN THE HOME HEALTH SETTING

Product Codes, Definitions, Allowables, & Product Examples: Group I Support Surfaces

HCPCS Code	Product Definition/Requirements	Reimbursed as a Rental/Purchase	2003 Medicare Part B Reimbursement Range	Product Examples*
FOAM				
E0199	Dry pressure pad for mattress - Base thickness of 2" or greater and peak height of 3" or greater for convoluted overlays. - 3" height or greater for nonconvoluted overlays. - Density that provides adequate pressure reduction. - Durable, waterproof cover.	Purchase	$27.24–$32.05	Mason Medical—Varizone II Span America—Geomatt™
E0184	Dry pressure mattress - Foam height of 5" or greater. - Density that provides adequate pressure reduction. - Durable, waterproof cover. - Can be placed directly on the bed frame.	Purchase	$165.50–$194.70	Invacare—CareGaurd 101™ B.G. Industries—Permafloat™ Gaymar—Top Gaurd II KCI—TheraRest™ Hill-Rom—SimpliMatt™
AIR				
E0197	Air pressure pad for mattress - Interconnected cells inflated with a pump. - Cell height of 3" or greater.	Purchase	$188.34–$221.58	EHOB—Waffle™ Gaymar™—Sof-Care Plus™ The ROHO Group—Prodigy Mattress Overlay
E0186	Air pressure mattress Interconnected cells inflated with a pump. - Cell height of 5" or greater. - Durable, waterproof cover. - Can be placed directly on a bed frame.	Rental	$17.26–$20.30	Atlantis Medical—Zaam Mattress
WATER				
E0198	Water pressure pad for mattress - Filled height of 3" or greater.	Purchase	$188.34–$221.58	Blue Chip Medical—Stat H2O Tempest International—Supra II Lotus Healthcare—Md3677 w/water
E0187	Water pressure mattress - Total height of 5" or greater. - Durable, waterproof cover. - Can be placed directly on the bed frame.	Rental	$19.73–$23.21	Flo Care—Flo
GEL				
E0185	Gel pressure pad for mattress - Gel height of 2" or greater.	Purchase	$271.88–$319.86	Blue Chip Medical—Stat Gel Lotus Healthcare—GL3666 (gel) Mason Medical—Sierra 3
E0196	Gel pressure mattress - Gel height of 5" or greater. - Durable, waterproof cover. - Can be placed directly on bed frame.	Rental	$27.62–$32.49	Grant—Dyna Soft
ALTERNATING PRESSURE				
E0180	Pressure pad, alternating with pump	Rental	$18.47–$21.73	Huntleigh—Alphabed™ Grant—Dyna Soft™ DuroMed Industries—Duro-matic APP & Pump
E0181	Pressure pad, alternating with pump, heavy duty - Air pump or blower that provides either sequential inlation or deflation of air cells or a low interface pressure through the overlay. - Inflated cell height of 2.5" or greater. - Provides adequate lift, reduces pressure, and prevents bottoming out.	Rental	$20.47–$24.08	

Wound, Ostomy and Continence Nurses Society ♦ 4700 W. Lake Avenue ♦ Glenview, IL 60025 ♦ www.wocn.org
* Product examples are included for reference only and are not intended to be all inclusive.
(page 2 of 4)

Fig. 1 (*continued*)

Challenges that lie ahead

Despite numerous research studies, the selection of the most appropriate support surface remains an arduous task for most clinicians. No single product stands out or is able to meet the needs of every patient, which creates further confusion and makes the decision-making process more

Professional Practice Fact Sheet | MEDICARE PART B COVERAGE FOR
SUPPORT SURFACES IN THE HOME HEALTH SETTING

Product Codes, Definitions, Allowables, & Product Examples: Group II Support Surfaces

HCPCS Code	Product Definition/Requirements	Reimbursed as a Rental/Purchase	2003 Medicare Part B Reimbursement Range	Product Examples*
NONPOWERED				
E0371	Nonpowered, advanced pressure-reducing overlay - Height and design of individual cells provides significantly more pressure reduction than a Group 1 overlay. - Prevents bottoming out - Total height of 3" or greater. - Surface designed to reduce friction and shear. - Evidence that the product is effective in treating conditions described by Group II coverage criteria.	Rental	$377.81–$444.48	ROHO—ROHO DRY FLOATATION™ Mattress System KCI—RIK Fluid Overlay™
E0373	Nonpowered, advanced pressure-reducing mattress - Height and design of individual cells provides significantly more pressure resuction than a Group I overlay. - Prevents bottoming out. - Total height of 5" or greater. - Surface designed to reduce friction and shear. - Evidence that the product is effective in treating conditions described by Group II coverage criteria. - Can be placed directly on a hospital bed frame.	Rental	$522.30–$614.47	KCI—RIK Fluid Mattress™ Span-America—Pressure Guard CFT™
POWERED				
E0372	Powered air overlay for mattress. - Air pump or blower which provides either sequential inflation and deflation or low interface pressure through the cells. - Inflated height of the air cells is 3.5" or greater. - Provides adequate lift, reduces pressure, and prevents bottoming out. - Surface that reduces friction and shear.	Rental	$458.44–$539.34	Plexus Medical—Air Express Hill-Rom—Acucair™ Huntleigh—Alpha Xcell KCI First Step Classic™
E0277	Alternating pressure mattress - Air pump or blower that provides either sequential inflation and deflation or low interface pressure through the cells. - Inflated height of the air cells is 5" or greater. - Provides adequate lift, reduces pressure, and prevents bottoming out. - Surface reduces friction and shear. - Can be placed directly on a bed frame.	Rental	$646.46–$759.36	Hill-Rom—Silkair™ KCI—First Step Tri-Cell™ Pegasus—Air Wave Therapeutic MRS™ Sen Tech Medical—Stage IV Invacare—MicroAir 3500S™ Huntleigh—DFS 2™ Air Care Therapy—Select Air
E0193	Powered air flotation bed - Semi-electric bed with a fully integrated powered pressure-reducing mattress. - Meets all of the requirements of E0277.	Rental	$767.94–$903.46	KCI—KinAir III

Wound, Ostomy and Continence Nurses Society ◆ 4700 W. Lake Avenue ◆ Glenview, IL 60025 ◆ www.wocn.org
Product examples are included for reference only and are not intended to be all inclusive.
(page 3 of 4)

Fig. 1 (*continued*)

complicated. Reimbursement for both useful and worthless products is another reason clinicians have difficulty in choosing the most appropriate and cost-effective surface for their patients. The National Pressure Ulcer Advisory Panel launched a 3-year initiative to develop standardized terminology, test methods, and reporting standards for support surfaces. The Support Surface Initiative was begun in January, 2002, and invited

Product Codes, Definitions, Allowables, & Product Examples: Group III Support Surfaces

HCPCS Code	Product Definition/Requirements	Reimbursed as a Rental/Purchase	2003 Medicare Part B Reimbursement Range	Product Examples*
NONPOWERED				
E0194	Air fluidized bed - A device employing the circulation of filtered air through silicone-coated ceramic beads creating the characteristics of fluid.	Rental	$2,766.19–$3,254.34	Hill-Rom—Clinitron™ KCI—Fluid Air HC™

Wound, Ostomy and Continence Nurses Society ◆ 4700 W. Lake Avenue ◆ Glenview, IL 60025 ◆ www.wocn.org
Product examples are included for reference only and are not intended to be all inclusive.
(page 4 of 4)

Fig. 1 (*continued*)

researchers, clinicians, scientists, policy makers, and manufacturers to develop support surface standards. The committee is also working with the European Pressure Ulcer Advisory Panel to establish international standards. The objective is not to rank each support surface, pitting one particular surface against another. Rather, the standards will facilitate

Table 2
Coverage and reimbursement of support surfaces across the care continuum

Care setting	Clinical coverage criteria	Reimbursement
Acute care	Per hospital coverage	Diagnostic-related groups
Skilled nursing facilities	Per facility protocol for Group I surfaces; Medicare Part B Support Surface Policy coverage criteria used as a guideline for Group II and III support surfaces	Medicare Part A (100 days); all routine and ancillary charges are under the Prospective Payment system
Long-term care (custodial care)	Per facility protocol; no agreed upon coverage criteria established	No reimbursement for support surfaces beyond Medicare Part A 100 skilled coverage days
Home health	Coverage criteria established per Medicare Part B Support Surface Policy	Medicare Part B; there are four Durable Medical Equipment Regional Carriers in the United States
Hospice	Per agency protocol	Per diem rate to cover all services and products provided; no extra money

defining performance characteristics and place them along a continuum to assist the clinician in making an informed choice [27].

Summary

The prevention and treatment of pressure ulcers are major concerns for health care providers across the care continuum. The selection of a support surface is an important component of a comprehensive pressure ulcer prevention program. The accepted standard in clinical practice for preventing pressure ulcers and other complications of immobility is to either turn patients manually at frequent intervals or to use a pressure-reducing device. The longer a patient is immobilized, the more profound will be the systemic complications. The costs associated with the complications of immobility are staggering in terms of human suffering, physiologic damage, and real dollars [28]. A variety of specialty beds, mattresses, and overlays have been designed to address pressure, shear, friction, and moisture. Limited data exist regarding the efficacy of these products. Clinicians want to choose a support surface for their patients on the basis of product performance. With the push toward establishing standards for testing methods and reporting information, clinicians can look forward to making support surface decisions based on the evidence and outcome data resulting from controlled clinical studies and expert opinion and consensus [29].

References

[1] Medical policy for pressure-reducing support surfaces by the Medicare part B Durable Medical Equipment Regional Carriers (DMERCs). Health Care Financing Administration; 1996.

[2] Armstrong D, Bortz P. An integrative review of pressure relief in surgical patients. AORN J 2001;73(3):645–8, 650–3.

[3] Centers for Disease Control. Injury research agenda–acute care: disability and rehabilitation. 2003. Available at: http://www.cdc.gov/ncipc/pub-res/research_agenda/10_acutecare.htm.

[4] Collins F, Hampton S. Use of Pressurease and airform mattresses in pressure ulcer care. Br J Nurs 2000;9(19):2104–8.

[5] Ferrell BA, Osterweil D, Christenson P. A randomized trial of low air-loss beds for treatment of pressure ulcers. JAMA 1993;269(4):494–7.

[6] Mayrovitz H, Regan MB, Larsen P. Effects of rhythmically alternating and static pressure support surfaces on skin microvascular perfusion. Wounds 1993;5(1):47–55.

[7] Agency for Health Care Research and Quality. Making health care safer: a critical analysis of patient safety practices: evidence report/technology assessment. Rockville (MD): US Department of Health and Human Services; 2001. p. 301–6.

[8] Conine TA, Hershler C. Effectiveness: a neglected dimension in the assessment of re-habilitation devices and equipment. Int J Rehabil Res 1991;14(2):117–22.

[9] van Rijswijk L. Evidence and support surfaces: an overview and analysis of the Blue Cross Blue Shield Technology Evaluation. 2000. p. 3–21.

[10] Cullum N, Deeks J, Sheldon TA, et al. Bed, mattresses and cushions for pressure sore prevention and treatment. The Cochrane Database of Systematic Reviews. Nov, 2001.

[11] Aronovitch SA. A comparative, randomized, controlled study to determine safety and efficacy of preventive pressure ulcer systems: preliminary analysis. Adv Wound Care 1998; 11(Suppl 3):S15–6.

[12] Nixon J, McElvenny D, Mason S, et al. A sequential randomized controlled trial using a double visco-elastic polymer pad and standard operating table mattress in the prevention of postoperative pressure sores. Int J Nurs Stud 1998;35:1932–3.

[13] Russell JA, Lichenstein SL. Randomized controlled trial to determine the safety and efficacy of a multi-cell pulsating dynamic mattress system in the prevention of pressure ulcers in patients undergoing cardiovascular surgery. Ostomy Wound Manage 2000;46:46–51, 54–5.

[14] Panel for the Prediction and Prevention of Pressure Ulcers in Adults. Pressure ulcers in adults: prediction and prevention. Clinical practice guideline, Number 3. Agency for Health Care Policy and Research, Public Health Service; 1992. Rockville (MD): US Department of Health and Human Services. AHCPR Publication #92–0047.

[15] Bergstrom N, Bennett MA, Carlson CE, et al. Treatment of pressure ulcers. Clinical practice guideline, Number 15. Agency for Health Care Policy and Research. 1994. Rockville (MD): US Department of Health and Human Services. AHCPR Publication #95–0653.

[16] Wound Ostomy & Continence Nurses Society. Guideline for prevention and management of pressure ulcers. Clinical practice guideline series No. 2. Glenview (IL): WOCN; 2003.

[17] Bates-Jensen BM. Pressure ulcers: pathophysiology and prevention. In: Sussman C, Bates-Jensen B, editors. Wound care: a collaborative practice manual for physical therapists and nurses. 1st edition. Gaithersburg (MD): Aspen; 1998. p. 241–5.

[18] Brienza DM, Geyer MJ, Sprigle S. Seating, positioning, and support surfaces. In: Baranoski S and Ayello EA, editors. Wound care essentials: Practice principles. Springhouse, PA: Lippincott, Williams & Wilkins; 2004, Chapter 11, p. 187–216.

[19] Whittemore R. Pressure-reduction support surfaces: a review of the literature. J Wound Ostomy Continence Nurs 1998;25(1):6–25.

[20] Fontaine R, Risley S, Castellino R. A quantitative analysis of pressure and shear in the effectiveness of support surfaces. J Wound Ostomy Continence Nurs 1998;25(5):233–9.

[21] Flam E. A new risk factor analysis. Ostomy Wound Manage 1991;33:28–31, 34.

[22] Reger S, Adams TC, Maklebust JA, et al. Validation test for climate control on air-loss supports. Arch Phys Med Rehabil 2001;82(5):597–603.

[23] Gutierrez A. Pressure lessons. Int J Rehab Res 2002;Dec:1–5.

[24] Pieper B. Mechanical forces: pressure, shear, and friction. In: Bryant RA, editor. Acute and chronic wounds: nursing management. St. Louis (MO): Mosby, 2000. p. 255–65.

[25] Fletcher J. Selecting pressure relieving equipment. J Wound Care 1995;4(6):2.

[26] Wells JA, Karr D. Interface pressure, wound healing, and satisfaction in the evaluation of a non-powered fluid mattress. Ostomy Wound Manage 1998;44(2):38–42, 44–6, 48.

[27] Fleck CA. Update on the NPUAP Support Surface Standards initiative. Extended Care Product News 2003;6–9.

[28] Melland HI, Langemo D, Hanson D, et al. Clinical evaluation of an automated turning bed. Orthop Nurs 1999;18(4):65–70.

[29] Krouskop T, van Rijwijk L. Standardizing performance-based criteria for support surfaces. Ostomy Wound Manage 1995;41(1):34–44.

ELSEVIER
SAUNDERS

Nurs Clin N Am 40 (2005) 267–279

NURSING
CLINICS
OF NORTH AMERICA

Facilitating Positive Outcomes in Older Adults with Wounds

Nancy A. Stotts, RN, EdD, FAAN[a],*,
Harriet W. Hopf, MD[b]

[a]School of Nursing, University of California San Francisco, 2 Koret Way, No. 631,
San Francisco, CA 94143, USA
[b]Department of Anesthesiology and Perioperative Care, University of California
San Francisco, San Francisco, CA 94143, USA

Older adults represent a significant portion of the wound care population. The number of individuals with wounds is anticipated to increase as the United States population ages. In 2002, 1 in every 12 Americans was at least 65 years of age, which totals approximately 35.6 million people. It is estimated that by 2030, this number will reach 71.5 million [1,2]. People who reach 65 years old have a life expectancy of an additional 18.1 years (19.4 for women and 16.4 for men). The population of oldest old, those 85 years of age or more, is increasing at the fastest rate and will increase to approximately 2.5% of the population by 2030 [2]. At that time, being more than 100 years old will be common, and we will have a large number of people in their 90s.

Older adults are different than younger people. More than 80% of seniors have at least one chronic condition, and 50% have at least two [3]. Additionally, they experience vision loss, hearing impairment, decreases in physical function, and alterations in cognition [4]. Although a small percentage of people live in long-term care facilities, most older adults live in the community. Their goal often is not to increase longevity but to have a good quality of life [5]. Women outlive men, and many women live alone. Between the ages of 65 and 74, approximately 13.8% of men and 30.6% of women live alone, whereas, beginning at age 75, 21.4% of men live alone, as do 49.4% of women [2]. The financial resources of many older people are constrained because they live longer than they had planned, and often, financial needs exceed their income. In fact, the income of more than half of

* Corresponding author.
E-mail address: nancy.stotts@nursing.ucsf.edu (N.A. Stotts).

0029-6465/05/$ - see front matter © 2005 Elsevier Inc. All rights reserved.
doi:10.1016/j.cnur.2004.09.005
nursing.theclinics.com

America's older people is severely limited; 31.5% live on $830 or less per month, and 21.4% receive between $830 and $1250 per month [1]. It is hard to imagine how older persons can stretch such a budget to include wound care costs.

The size of the population of older adults with wounds is difficult to estimate. Of the 41 million surgical procedures performed in the United States, 36% of them are performed on person 65 and older [6]. All of these individuals experience healing needs. Diabetes is present in 8.6 million persons who are 60 years of age or older [7]. Approximately 15% to 20% of persons with diabetes will be hospitalized for a diabetes-related wound in their lifetime [8]. Venous disease is seen in approximately 2% of the population, and although venous disease often begins in younger persons, the prevalence peaks at age 60 to 80 [9]. New onset pressure ulcers are estimated to occur in up to 29% of long-term care patients [10], and the incidence in acute care is variable, occurring in 5% of blacks and 15% of whites, in a large multisite study [11]. Thus, there are significant wound care needs among older people.

When possible, health care professionals expect the older person with a wound to understand wound care issues, participate in decisions about wound care, as well as all aspects of their physical care, and, if the wound is located in an accessible area, to actually perform their wound care. Their participation is modulated by a number of factors, including their ability to understand instructions and make decisions, their physical capacity for self-care, and their personal goals and how important the wound care is in their overall life, and whether they are receiving care in the hospital, a long-term care facility, or the home. Consideration also must be given to whether the wound is able to heal, how to maximize quality of life, and to balancing aggressive wound care with palliation. When the patient is unable to make decisions, understand the plan, or perform the wound care, then the expectation is that the family or designated decision maker will participate in wound care-related planning and implementation.

The expectations that older people will understand wound care issues and choices of treatment available to them, and participate in wound care decisions and physical care as well as have personal goals for their life are not different than for younger individuals. Yet physiologic changes associated with aging require health professionals to consider additional parameters. Older persons heal at a slower rate and are at increased risk of infection and dehiscence. Their understanding of wound-related issues may be modulated by decreased sensory ability, for example, loss of hearing and decreased vision. Information processing may be impaired because of temporary or permanent cognitive changes. Alterations in functional status may limit wound self-care. Most care is driven by an individual clinician's experience, because research in this area is sparse. Application of existing knowledge about older persons specifically to the care of wounds is limited.

This article focuses on knowledge needed to care for older persons with wounds. We briefly examine literature on the type of wound healing problems older adults experience, and then major changes in sensory processes, cognition, and functional status in older patients will be described. Approaches will be interspersed to assess and address sensory loss, cognitive and functional status as they affect wound care. Examples of use of this knowledge in clinical care are found in the boxes throughout the text.

Healing in the older adult

Aging affects all phases of healing, independent of the increased rate of comorbidities that may themselves impair healing. The sum of these changes is slower healing [12], which is true of both acute (surgical or traumatic) and chronic wounds (venous ulcers, diabetic ulcers, and pressure ulcers). Older persons may develop chronic wounds more frequently because of delayed acute healing, and chronic wounds that heal more slowly are at increased risk of secondary complications such as infection [13].

A number of changes are known or thought to occur with age, although much is not yet known. Skin morphology changes, with a decrease in dermal thickness and the absolute number of cells, flattening of the dermoepidermal junction, and decreased collagen and proteoglycan content compared with younger skin [14–16]. Immune cells, including neutrophils and macrophages, demonstrate decreased migration, phagocytosis, respiratory burst, and growth factor production [17–20].

Keratinocytes demonstrate decreased rates of migration, thus delaying epithelization [21]. Growth factor levels and the response to growth factors are generally decreased in the wounds of older patients [22,23]. These changes are seen even in healthy older volunteers, thus demonstrating that wound healing impairment in older individuals cannot be attributed solely to the increase in comorbidities. Older patients undergoing major abdominal surgery demonstrate a decreased capacity to lay down collagen tissue [24]. However, some of the changes that are seen with aging are reversible or potentially reversible. Ashcroft et al [25] demonstrated that hormone replacement therapy (with estrogen) in older normal volunteers increased healing capacity in a test wound. Papadakis et al [23] demonstrated that the correction of age related insulin-like growth factor-1 deficiency with low-dose growth hormone resulted in increased healing capacity in aged men.

Another area in which aging may impair wound healing is through increased susceptibility to infection. Mangram et al [26] compiled published data on prevention of surgical site infection, previously known as wound infection. Although age is listed as a patient characteristic that may influence the risk of surgical site infection development, no literature is cited as supporting its inclusion, and none of the recommendations specifically address older persons. Other data do indicate increased infection rate in older surgical patients [27,28] and indicate that decreased humoral and cell-mediated immune response occur with old age that is compounded by the immune impairment seen with concomitant disease [29].

It is important to recognize that the presentation of wound infection in older persons is atypical. The presentation may involve an entirely different body system [4] and include changes in mental status, alterations in functional status, reports of pain, or complaints of malaise, rather than the typical combination of fever, increased white blood cell count, and inflammation at the wound site.

Another problem that occurs at a greater rate in older than in younger persons is dehiscence. Dehiscence increases the risk of infection as well as the length of hospitalization and recovery time. One study [30] found that the tensile strength of incisions is less in older rats than in younger, and the risk of dehiscence in older rats is greater. In a review that examined the rate of dehiscence in surgical patients, Carlson [31] showed that the incidence of dehiscence before 1940 was approximately 0.4%, and from 1950 to 1984 the rate was approximately 0.59%. Studies performed after 1985 show a dehiscence rate of approximately 1.2%. Although it may appear that the incidence is increasing, data are only available from published studies, and not all dehiscence data are published, so this may be an underestimation of the problem. It also is important to recognize that researchers who report dehiscence data do not control for comorbidities, which may confound the effect of age on dehiscence.

Of importance to clinical practice is the issue of when dehiscence occurs. Carlson [31] reports that the average period is postoperative day 7, recognizing that the range is from 1 to more than 21 days. Serosanguinous drainage that occurs more than 48 hours after wound closure is seen in some cases before dehiscence and so can be regarded as a sign of impending dehiscence. In addition, the lack of a healing ridge on postoperative day 5 has been identified in one prospective study [32] as an additional sign of impending dehiscence (Box 1).

Sensory losses

Hearing

Defects in the sensory system, that is, hearing and seeing, interfere with patients' ability to understand the decisions related to wound care management and to participate meaningfully in their care. Patients with hearing loss may not be able to understand instructions for wound care and therefore may not be able to perform self-care.

Sensory loss is common in the elderly. In a population of community-dwelling older people who were followed longitudinally, mild hearing impairment was seen in approximately 30% of people during their 50s. Moderate or greater hearing loss increased with age (14.9% in the 60s, 23.6% in the 70s, and 34.6% in the 80s and greater). In addition, men had

---

Box 1. Healing in older adults

Mr. Paul is a 76-year-old man with a 40-year history of insulin-dependent diabetes and bilateral Charcot foot. He underwent amputation of the first three toes of his right foot 8 days ago. During his first postoperative visit, the clinic nurse noted that his foot incision site was clean and well approximated with sutures. There was no erythema or swelling. However, a moderate amount of serosanguinous drainage was present along 2 cm of the lateral aspect of the incision line. This finding suggests that Mr. Paul is at risk for dehiscence.

---

more severe average impairment than women [33]. Functional impairment in this study was related to the degree of hearing impairment.

Often, the elderly can hear sound but the words are indistinct, and they cannot decode specific words. They lose high-pitched sounds and the ability to discriminate between words when speech is rapid, and cannot differentiate speech from background noise [34]. The accumulation of these losses results in words becoming distorted and difficult to understand. Instructions for wound care cannot be followed if they are not understood.

Lyons et al [4] recommends screening for hearing loss with the whisper test because its sensitivity and specificity are in the 70% to 100% range. The whisper test takes less than 1 minute to perform, and it requires no equipment. It is performed in a quiet environment and with the patient alone. Family members are asked to step out of the examination area because they may inadvertently cue the patient, and having an acknowledged hearing loss may be embarrassing to the patient. The test is performed by having the patient occlude the ear that is not being tested. The examiner covers his or her lips with the hand and whispers so that the patient cannot lip-read. The examiner, located 1 to 2 feet from the patient's ear, whispers a two-syllable word (eg, "18") toward the unoccluded ear with approximately equal emphasis on each syllable [35].

When the patient has a hearing aid, it is important that it be in place, turned on, and has working batteries. Having a hearing aid does not guarantee that the patient can hear because background noise is amplified by the hearing aid and may interfere with the patient's understanding of what is being communicated.

Loss of hearing has significant implications for the nurse providing wound care. Recognizing that the patient has a hearing loss will allow the professional to take measures to enhance communication. The professional caring for the patient should talk with the individual in a quiet place, with minimal background noise. This means that a radio or television, if present, needs to be turned off. The health care provider should get the person's attention and stand directly in front of him or her when talking so that lip reading can take place. Using a loud voice, the health care provider should speak clearly and slowly to enhance understanding [34]. Asking the patient to summarize what has been said is one method to validate that information was heard and processed.

Vision

Overall vision changes begin early, with a loss of near vision that begins at approximately age 40. With the Alameda study data [33], approximately half of the population shows a vision loss by age 60, and the percentage of persons with vision loss increases with age, as does the severity. In the 60- to 69-year-old age group, 41.4% had mild vision impairment, and 8.7% had moderate or greater impairment. By age 80 or greater, 33.8% had mild vision impairment, and 29.8% had moderate or greater impairment.

Simple screening can be done with a Snellen chart [4]. There are a number of common vision pathologies in the elderly, for example, cataracts, glaucoma, and macular degeneration, and each condition requires referral to an ophthalmologist for evaluation and treatment.

Vision is important in the care of wound patients because it allows the patient to evaluate changes in wound condition and understand written instructions and is critical to direct manipulation of the dressing. Vision is critical to evaluating wound healing: it allows patients to see the difference between a healing wound and an infected wound and to identify any abnormal wound drainage, slough, or necrotic tissue. Box 2 illustrates the situation of an older adult with sensory changes.

Box 2. Sensory changes

Mrs. Y is an 80-year-old woman who was admitted to long-term care 2 weeks ago. She experienced a recent cerebrovascular accident, with left-sided hemiplegia, and developed a stage III sacral ulcer while hospitalized. She is able to do very little for herself. She becomes combative every time her sacral dressing is changed. She does not seem to comprehend what the nurses are doing. One of the nurses reviewed Mrs. Y's admission Minimal Data Set data and found that the patient had no cognitive deficit, but she uses both a hearing aid and glasses. On exploration, the nurse located them in a bag in the patient's closet. When the hearing aid and glasses were given to Mrs. Y, she was able to put them on. The nurse explained about the needed sacral ulcer care, and the patient was cooperative during her wound care and seemed better able to participate in self-care activities.

Although not a vision issue, when written materials are used, the reading ability of the individual is considered and whether cartoon pictures or words should be used to communicate the message [36]. Regardless of which method is used, a vision-related issue is the color of the lettering and its background. Older persons have more trouble differentiating between blues and greens than between reds and yellows; thus, reds and yellows should be used more frequently in pictures and written materials. In addition, black lettering on white background is easier for older people to decode than green lettering on yellow paper.

Print type size is also important, and the use of 14- or 16-point font size is indicated when working with older people [37]. Ideally, the clinician should provide large print black letters on white paper and present the content in a well-lighted area. Older people also need sufficient time to read and understand the material presented.

Cognitive status

Cognitive capacity is an individual's ability to perceive, register, store, retrieve, and use information [38] and is measured many ways. Some measurements are one-dimensional, and others combine several aspects. The instruments vary in the amount of education required by the examiner before their use, the amount of time required to administer them, and where they can be used (ie, bedside or clinic).

Cognitive changes are often unrecognized by nurses. In a study [39] of nearly 800 adults 70 years of age or older, nurses performed routine assessment and compared their evaluation with researchers' evaluation using a standardized tool. Delirium occurred in 16% of patients, and nurses identified it somewhat more than 30% of the time. Four risk factors for under-recognition were identified: hypoactive delirium, being 80 years old or greater, vision impairment, and dementia. Standardized cognitive assessment would help mitigate this problem.

Of interest in working with a patient with a wound is a global measure of cognition that can be administered rapidly and provides information about the individual's ability to participate in their care decisions and physically treat the wound. A number of global measures exist. Two common instruments are the Mental Status Questionnaire (MSQ) [40] and the Mini-Mental State Examination (MMSE) [41].

The MSQ is a 10-item scale that was designed to measure cognitive function in the elderly. Errors scored from 1 to 2 indicate an insignificant problem, 3 to 5 a moderate impairment, and 6 to 10 a moderate to severe impairment. The MSQ was an early cognitive screening tool and has been criticized because of the lack of theoretical justification for items [42]. A strength of this instrument is that it is easy to administer and completed quickly, and answers to the questions are verifiable. Items on the MSQ assess a patient's orientation to place and location, knowledge of birth and current year and month, and the name of the presidents. An example of an MSQ item is "What is the month now?" Testing with this instrument does not rely on the patient's mathematical ability to receive a score that reflects high cognitive functioning.

The MMSE addresses short- and long-term memory, orientation, attention, calculation, registration, language, praxis, and copying of a design [41]. It is composed of 11 items. Each item is given a score, and the total is 30. A score of less than 24 indicates cognitive impairment [41,43]. The MMSE is considered a brief screening tool and is not to be used as a diagnosis of dementia [44]. An experienced clinician can administer the instrument in 5 to 10 minutes. An example of an MSSE item is "Please repeat the following three words (shirt, brown, honesty)" [41]. Box 3 provides an example of a patient demonstrating cognitive changes.

Functional status

Functional status is generally considered a measure of physical health or function. The ability to perform self-care activities depends on functional status. The ability to care for a wound depends on both gross and fine motor activity. Gross motor activities include gathering supplies and dressing materials, showering, and cleansing the wound. Fine motor activities include removal of old dressings, application of topical agents, and redressing the wound.

Generally, functional status includes dimensions of activities, instrumental activities, and advanced activities of daily living. Activities of daily living

---

Box 3. Cognitive changes

Mr. A is a 73-year-old man who was admitted to the hospital 4 days ago for acute respiratory failure secondary to pneumonia. On the day of discharge, his venous ulcer dressing on the left lateral malleolus was changed and wrapped with a 4-layer bandage. The nurse reviewed his wound care with him. When the nurse finished the teaching, Mr. A asked again why his leg was bandaged. The nurse explained again but could not quite understand why the patient asked the question. She reviewed the chart and found that there was no documentation of cognitive assessment at admission because it had been deferred owing to his acute respiratory failure. The nurse used the MMSE to assess Mr. A's cognitive state and discovered major cognitive defects. She re-evaluated the discharge plan and mobilized the wife, physician, and social worker to have an interdisciplinary team meeting with the patient present.

are self-care activities. Instrumental activities of daily living are more complex activities associated with independent living such as shopping or balancing a checkbook. Advanced activities of daily living contribute to quality of life and include recreation (eg, playing bridge or golf) and community activities.

Well-established instruments that will be discussed here are the index of independence in activities of daily living [45] and the Medical Outcomes Study Physical Functioning Measure [46]. Other scales include the Barthel Index [47], which is used to measure functional independence and mobility in the chronically ill. The Functional Status Independence Measure [48], which measures functional and cognitive disability, often is used in rehabilitation settings.

Katz' scale [45] is probably the test most often used with the elderly [49]. It is an ordinal scale that rates six activities of daily living functions, including bathing, dressing, going to the toilet, transferring from bed to chair, continence, and feeding. One strength of the scale is that it is a Likert scale in which gradations of function can be assessed. For example, independence in dressing includes the ability of the elderly person to take their clothes from the closet or drawer, put them on, and fasten them. It includes putting on braces if the individual wears them. Partial independence is present if the person can perform everything except tie their shoes. A person who needs help in getting their clothes or putting them on or one who does not dress, or who only partially dresses is considered dependent [50].

The Older Americans Resource and Services Center instrument is a multidimensional instrument that has established validity and reliability across settings. One subscale addresses physical functioning. The physical functioning scale includes data on activities of daily living as well as instrumental activities of daily living. This scale has been adapted for use in various settings and is widely used in research. Box 4 is a clinical example of community-dwelling older adult for whom functional limitations affect her self-care ability.

Summary

Older people with wounds are not the same as younger people with wounds. Older people experience biologic differences in wound healing that result in delayed healing, increased wound infection, and a greater incidence of dehiscence. Clinicians need to assess the risk of dehiscence in the older population, looking for serous drainage from the incision line and the absence of a palpable healing ridge.

It is critical to recognize that older persons' presentation of wound infection is atypical. More subtle signs such as alteration in cognitive status and changes in function may indicate the presence of infection. The clinician who cares for older persons must be an exquisite detective when such changes occur to identify the source of the problem.

Box 4. Functional changes

Ms. H is a 90-year-old woman who lives alone. She underwent
  bilateral hip replacement, and the last surgery was performed
  5 years ago. Recently, she traumatized her left calf and now
  has a wound that is 3 cm × 4 cm. The plan is for her to
  change the dressing twice per week and for a home health
  nurse to change the dressing once per week. Ms. H is able
  to perform her own cooking, toileting, and transfer. She had
  some trouble getting dressed because of her arthritis, and
  she had modified her wardrobe to include pants with an
  elastic waist, pull-on blouses, and Velcro-shoes. A full
  assessment of sensory, functional, and cognitive status by
  the home health nurse revealed that functional changes
  were Ms. H's primary limits. The home health nurse concluded
  that Ms. H was unable to change her own dressing because
  of a lack of fine motor movement resulting from her arthritis.
  The nurse conferred with Ms. H's physician, and together
  they developed a plan that used a dressing that required
  changing only once per week and that would be done by
  the home health nurse. At the same time, the nurse would
  monitor the healing of Ms. H's wound.

As part of the normal trajectory of aging, older persons experience
sensory loss and so may require accommodation when explanations are
given to them about their wound and their wound care choices. Health care
providers must consider hearing and vision changes that occur in older
adults and tailor their explanations and teaching so that the message reaches
the older adult and is successfully processed.

Older persons have a higher incidence of cognitive changes and
functional decline than do their younger counterparts, and these changes
need to be assessed before a plan of care is developed to care for the older
person with a wound. Limited data are available to help the clinician know
the cognitive and functional level that is critical for older persons to
understand their wound care choices, perform their own wound care, and to
make choices about who will provide the care if they are unable to perform
self-care. These seemingly basic issues raise questions for clinicians as we
strive to provide evidence-based care to this ever-increasing population of
older Americans.

References

[1] Administration on Aging. A profile of older Americans. 2003. Washington, DC: US
    Department of Health and Human Services, 2003. p. 1–3.

[2] Centers for Disease Control and Prevention. Older person's health. April 12, 2004. Available at: www.cdc.gov/nchs/fastats/older-americans/htm. Accessed April 12, 2004.

[3] Centers for Disease Control and Prevention. Healthy aging: Preventing disease and improving quality of life among older Americans. Available at: www.cdc.gov/aging. Accessed April 10, 2004.

[4] Lyons WL, Johnston CB, Covinsky KE, et al. Geriatric medicine. In: Tierney LM Jr, McPhee SJ, Papadakis MA, editors. Current medical diagnosis and treatment. New York: Lange Medical Books; 2001. p. 44–63.

[5] Alliance for Aging Research. Medical never-never land: ten reasons why America is not ready for the coming age boom. February, 2002. http://www.agingresearch.org/brochures/nevernever/welcome.html. Accessed January 2, 2003.

[6] Hall MJ, DeFrances CJ. 2001 National hospital discharge survey. advance data. Centers for Disease Control and Prevention 2003;332:1–6.

[7] American Diabetes Association. National diabetes fact sheet. April 10, 2004. Available at: http://www.diabetes.org/diabetes-statistics/national-diabetes-fact-sheet.jsp. Accessed April 10, 2004.

[8] Reiber GE, Boyko EJ, Smith DG. Lower extremity foot ulcers and amputations in diabetes. In: National Diabetes Data Group (US). Diabetes in America. 2nd edition. Bethesda (MD): National Institute of Diabetes and Digestive and Kidney Diseases; 1995.

[9] Callam MJ, Harper DR, Dale JJ, et al. Chronic ulcer of the leg: clinical history. BMJ 1986; 294:1389–91.

[10] Horn SD, Bender SA, Ferguson ML, et al. The National Pressure Ulcer Long-Term Care study: Pressure ulcer development in long term care residents. J Am Geriatr Soc 2004;52(3): 359–67.

[11] Bergstrom N, Braden BJ. Predictive validity of the Braden scale among black and white subjects. Nurs Res 2002;51(6):398–403.

[12] Brem H, Tomic-Canic M, Tarnovskata A, et al. Healing of elderly patients with diabetic foot ulcers, venous stasis ulcers and pressure ulcers. Surg Technol Int 2003;11:161–7.

[13] Livesley NJ, Chow AW. Infected pressure ulcers in elderly individuals. Clin Infect Dis 2002; 35:1390–6.

[14] Fenske NA, Lober CW. Structural and functional changes of normal aging skin. J Am Acad Dermatol 1986;15:571–85.

[15] Kurban RS, Bhawan J. Histologic changes in skin associated with aging. J Dermatol Surg Oncol 1990;16:908–14.

[16] Montagna W, Carlisle K. Structural changes in ageing skin. Br J Dermatol 1990;122(Suppl 35):S61–70.

[17] Lipschitz DA, Udupa KB. Influence of aging and protein deficiency on neutrophil function. J Gerontol 1986;41:690–4.

[18] Ashcroft GS, Horan MA, Ferguson MW. Aging is associated with reduced deposition of specific extracellular matrix components, an upregulation of angiogenesis, and an altered inflammatory response in a murine incisional wound healing model. J Invest Dermatol 1997; 108:430–7.

[19] Ashcroft GS, Horan MA, Ferguson MW. The effects of ageing on immunocalisation of growth factors and their receptors in a murine incisional model. J Anat 1997;190: 351–65.

[20] Ashcroft GS, Horan MA, Ferguson MW. Aging alters the inflammatory and endothelial cell adhesion molecule profiles during human cutaneous wound healing. Lab Invest 1998;78(1): 47–58.

[21] Svedman P, Svedman C, Njalsson T. Epithelialization and blood flow in suction blister wounds on healthy volunteers. J Invest Surg 1991;4:175–89.

[22] Xia YP, Zhao Y, Tyrone JW, et al. Differential activation of migration by hypoxia in keratinocytes isolated from donors of increasing age: implication for chronic wounds in the elderly. J Invest Dermatol 2001;116:50–6.

[23] Papadakis MA, Hamon G, Stotts N, et al. Effect of growth hormone replacement on wound healing in healthy older men. Wound Repair Regen 1996;4:421–5.

[24] Lenhardt R, Hopf HW, Marker E, et al. Perioperative collagen deposition in elderly and young men and women. Arch Surg 2000;135:71–4.

[25] Ashcroft GS, Mills SJ, Ashworth JJ. Ageing and wound healing. Biogerontology 2002;3: 337–45.

[26] Mangram AJ, Horan TC, Pearson ML, et al. for the Centers for Disease Control and Prevention Hospital Infection Control Practices Advisory Committee. Guideline for prevention of surgical site infection, 1999. Am J Infect Control 1999;27(2):9–132.

[27] Nieto A, Lozano M, Moro MT, et al. Determinants of wound infections after surgery for breast cancer. Zentralbl Gynakol 2002;128:429–33.

[28] Peivandi AA, Kasper-Konig W, Quinkenstein E, et al. Risk factors influencing the outcome after surgical treatment of complicated deep sternal wound complications. Cardiovasc Surg 2003;11(3):207–12.

[29] Esposito S. Immune system and surgical site infection. J Chemother 2001;12:12–6.

[30] Goodson WH III, Hunt TK. Wound healing and aging. J Invest Derm 1979;73(1):88–91.

[31] Carlson MA. Acute wound failure. Surg Clin North Am 1997;77(3):607–36.

[32] Pareira MD, Serkes KD. Prediction of wound disruption by use of the healing ridge. Surg Gynecol Obstet 1962;115:72–4.

[33] Wallhagen MI, Strawbridge WJ, Shema SJ, et al. Comparative impact of healing and vision impairment on subsequent functioning. JAGS 2001;49:1086–92.

[34] Raisin JH. Measurement issues with the elderly. In: Frank-Stromborg M, Olsen SL, editors. Instruments for clinical health-care research. 3rd edition. Boston: Jones & Bartlett Publishers; 2004. p. 47–55.

[35] Siedel HM, Ball JW, Dains JE, et al, editors. Mosby's guide to physical examination. 5th edition. St. Louis (MO): Mosby; 2003. p. 330–3.

[36] Weinrich SP, Boyd MD, Herman J. Tool adaptation to reduce health disparities. In: Frank-Stromborg M, Olsen SL, editors. Instruments for clinical health-care research. 3rd edition. Boston: Jones & Bartlett Publishers; 2004. p. 20–30.

[37] Weinrich SP, Boyd M, Nussbaum J. Continuing education: adapting strategies to teach the elderly. J Gerontol Nurs 1989;15:17–21.

[38] Foreman MD, Fletcher K, Mion LC, et al. Assessing cognitive function. In: Mezy MD, Fulmer T, Abraham I, editors. Geriatric nursing protocols for best practice. 2nd edition. New York: Springer; 2003. p. 99–115.

[39] Inouye SK, Foreman MD, Mion LC, et al. Nurses' recognition of delirium and its symptoms: comparison of nurse and researcher ratings. Arch Intern Med 2001;161(20): 2467–73.

[40] Kahn RL, Goldfarb AL, Pollack M, et al. Brief objective measures for the determination of mental status in the aged. Am J Psychiatry 1960;117:326–8.

[41] Folstein M, Folstein S, McHugh P. Mini-mental state examination: a practical guide for grading the cognitive state of patients for clinicians. J Psychiatr Res 1975;12(3):189–98.

[42] McDowell I, Newell C. Mental status testing. In: McDowell I, Newell C, editors. Measuring health. A guide to rating scales and questionnaires. New York: Oxford University Press; 1966. p. 308–11.

[43] Cella D, Nowinski CJ. Measuring quality of life in chronic illness: the functional assessment of chronic illness therapy measurement system. Arch Phys Med Rehabil 2002;83(Suppl 2): S10–7.

[44] Tombaugh TN, McIntyre NJ. The mini-mental state examination: a comprehensive review. JAGS 1992;40(9):922–35.

[45] Katz S, Ford AB, Moskowitz RW, et al. Studies of illness in the aged. the Index of ADL: a standardized measure of biological and psychosocial function. JAMA 1963;185:914–9.

[46] Ernst M, Ernst NS. Functional capacity. In: Mangen DJ, Peterson WA, editors. Research instruments in social gerontology. vol. 3. Minneapolis (MN): University of Minneapolis Press; 1984. p. 9–84.

[47] Mahoney FL, Barthel DW. Functional evaluation: the Barthel index. Md State Med J 1965; 14:61–5.

[48] Granger CV, Cotter AC, Hamilton BB, et al. Functional assessment scales: a study of persons with multiple sclerosis. Arch Phys Med Rehabil 1990;7(11):870–5.

[49] Kresevic DM, Mezey M. Assessment of function. In: Mezey M, Fulmer T, Abraham I, Zwicker D, editors. Geriatric nursing protocols for best practice. 2nd edition. New York: Springer; 2003. p. 31–46.

[50] Sehy YB, Williams MP. Functional assessment. In: Stone JT, Wyman JF, Salisbury SA, editors. Clinical gerontological nursing: a guide to advanced practice. 2nd edition. Philadelphia: WB Saunders; 1999. p. 175–99.

ELSEVIER
SAUNDERS

NURSING
CLINICS
OF NORTH AMERICA

Nurs Clin N Am 40 (2005) 281–294

Wound Care at End of Life

Stephanie Myers Schim, PhD, RN,
CNAA, APRN, BC[a],*,
Bernadette Cullen, MSN, RN, CWOCN[b]

[a]College of Nursing, Wayne State University, Detroit, MI 48202, USA
[b]Acute/Post Acute Nursing Services, East Jefferson General Hospital, Metairie, LA, USA

Currently there is a large amount of interest in improving end-of-life (EOL) care in the United States. This interest is spurred, in part, by the "graying of America" [1] as more people extend their life spans into "old old age." Aging of the demographic population bulge called the "baby boomer" generation also contributes to the increased interest. Baby boomers, now in positions of authority in government and health care sectors, are taking care of their elderly parents and experiencing firsthand many of the problems of existing end-of-life approaches. Boomers are also now facing their own looming old age and the realities of their own mortality. It is agreed that the traditional Western health care system needs to make significant changes in the way death is regarded and how the dying are treated. Nurses and other members of the interdisciplinary health care team need to be educated for end-of-life care excellence [2]. Quality end-of-life care is recognized as an essential component of quality of life. Support continues to grow for the fundamental belief of hospice and palliative care that all people have the right to die with dignity. To achieve a level of care consistent with this belief, patients and families must be an integral part of the plan of care. Patient and family goals are central concerns for professional nursing.

This article focuses on the integration of end-of-life concepts with currently accepted wound care principles. Juxtaposition of concepts and methods from EOL and wound care perspectives is critical to the professional nurse's management of patient and family care at one of the most significant transition points in the human experience.

* Corresponding author.
   E-mail address: s.schim@wayne.edu (S.M. Schim).

Care of chronic wounds with the terminally ill patient

The care of chronic wounds presents nursing challenges with any type of patient; however, unique concerns exist with the terminal care patient population. Development of chronic wounds at the end of life has been clearly documented in the literature. It has been noted by researchers [3] in the United Kingdom that 26% of patients admitted to one inpatient palliative care unit had pressure ulcers on admission, and another 12% of patients developed ulcers during their inpatient stay. Review of the literature further reveals little evidence regarding prevalence and incidence data for end-of-life wounds in the hospice setting, minimal standardization for pressure ulcer care, and broad acknowledgment of the pain and suffering associated with pressure ulcers. Among others, Hanson et al [4] have articulated the need to adapt existing pressure ulcer protocols for patients approaching the end of life.

The principal goals for palliative wound therapy are symptom management and improvement of quality of life. To achieve these goals, the key points of wound care are to maintain optimal skin integrity, keep the patient as comfortable as possible, manage incontinence, and support the caregiver. Palliative wound care components include controlling pain and odor, managing exudates, and minimizing dressing changes [5,6].

Chronic wound care covers many types of wounds, including pressure ulcers, venous or arterial ulcers, wounds resulting from trauma or surgery, and diabetic ulcers. Management issues with regard to planning care are similar for these wound types. The basic care directives include following evidence-based wound care principles, understanding the cause of the wound, intervening when appropriate, and integrating care with comfort initiatives. This article focuses on pressure ulcer management because this is the most commonly encountered wound and provides the exemplar for the care of chronic wounds at end of life.

End-of-life trajectories

Four patterns, or trajectories, have been identified and widely applied in the EOL literature. Although every death is unique in many ways, conceptualizing commonalities has proved useful since the patterns were originally described by Glaser and Strauss [7]. Brief descriptions of each pattern and the attendant wound care issues are provided here.

In the sudden death trajectory, a person is living in a relatively good state of health and functions at a high level of activity of daily living, and death occurs quickly and often unexpectedly. Many times, the proximal cause of death is a wound or wounds from a knife, gun, or motor vehicle accident. Wounds associated with loss of life are usually associated with massive trauma or damage to vital organs that make the injury incompatible with life. In other instances there are no wounds associated with the cause of death. Heart attack, stroke, and many sudden onset communicable disease infections are examples of sudden death without wound issues.

In the chronic disease trajectory, a person develops a chronic disease that causes some limitation of function compared with the premorbid state. Over time, there are exacerbations and remissions in the patient's condition. After each episode of acute illness, the person returns to a level of health and function that is slightly lower than was experienced before the exacerbation. Examples of chronic diseases are diabetes mellitus and HIV/AIDS. Both of these conditions, and many others that conform to the chronic disease trajectory pattern, are also associated with chronic wound problems.

Along the organ failure trajectory, the person progresses from a relatively healthy state and a high level of functional ability to death over a period of time. The pattern is characterized by a marked decline in function and the absence of major remissions. The period from diagnosis to death may be a few days, weeks, months, or even years, but the decline is steady, and the end is sure. This trajectory is the common pattern for incurable cancers and is sometimes referred to as "the cancer model." Much of the work in end-of-life care has been performed using this pattern as the prime exemplar.

On the frailty trajectory, a person enters the last phase of life in a state of overall poor health and slowly declines from that state. The frailty pattern is often associated with persons of advanced old age who have been in robust health earlier in their lives and are now dwindling in function and strength. This pattern often describes the demise of patients with Alzheimer's disease and those who simply die of old age. General frailty and increasingly frail skin often combine with decreased mobility, hydration, and nutrition to put persons on this trajectory at high risk for wounds.

Concepts of palliative care

The National Hospice and Palliative Care Organization defines palliative care as treatment that enhances comfort and improves the quality of an individual's life during the last phase of life. No specific therapy is excluded from consideration. The test of palliative care lies in the agreement among the individual, physicians, primary caregiver, and the hospice team that the expected outcome is relief from distressing symptoms and the easing of pain or enhancing quality of life. The decision to intervene with active palliative care is based on an ability to meet stated goals rather than affect the underlying disease. The individual's choices and decisions regarding care are paramount and must be followed [8].

Once considered to be mutually exclusive approaches, there is growing recognition of a complementary relationship between traditional curative care and palliative care. At the initial diagnosis, the entire emphasis is often placed on medical and surgical treatments to produce a cure. Over time, as treatments are tried and prognosis is reassessed, the focus of effort gradually shifts away from cure toward more palliative efforts. There may not be a single point in time when the focus of effort shifts to palliation or comfort care. Providers, patients, and family members may make the transition gradually. As knowledge and acceptance of palliative care principles become more widespread, attention to patient comfort, management of symptom distress, and appropriate pain control are more widely acknowledged.

Hospice programs have provided much of the leadership in the area of palliative care, but hospice enrollment requires that patients have a prognosis of less than 6 months and have given up all treatment before enrollment. These limitations have been recognized as barriers for many patients and families. Hospice programs have embraced the concepts of palliative care to expand their repertoire of services. In addition, nonhospice settings such as hospitals and nursing homes have begun to include more palliative care approaches.

Family involvement in wound care at end of life

Patient and caregiver are frequently identified as one unit in hospice and palliative care contexts. Hospice care is covered under Medicare, Medicaid, most private insurance plans, and through managed care companies. As the majority of hospice patients are receiving Medicare hospice benefits [9], it is reasonable to infer that many are cared for by similarly aged spouses or by adult children (usually daughters). Health care professionals need to synthesize accepted wound care and end-of-life principles that will support the wishes of both the dying patient and the family. Two conditions in which this is particularly important are pressure ulcers and pain management.

Family caregivers seem to have particular difficulty dealing with pressure ulcers because many believe that pressure ulcers are signs of neglect. This belief may add guilt and embarrassment to an already burdened family caring for a dying person at home. It may also lead to dissatisfaction and potential legal action on the part of families with someone dying in an institutional setting. Nurses and other health care professionals need to assist families in understanding the causes of pressure ulcers and the common occurrence of ulcers among terminally ill patients.

Family caregivers also may have difficulty with patient pain and pain management protocols. Many patients and family members live in fear of uncontrolled pain at the end of life, but many also have fears about perceived over-medication and possible addiction. Nursing responsibilities include the assessment of pain and intervention to decrease or eliminate pain and suffering. EOL wound management presents an additional potential source of discomfort and challenges pain assessment and intervention skills. Patients and family members may need to be educated about current pain relief protocols and may need to have their fears about addiction and respiratory suppression addressed. They may also benefit greatly from suggestions and demonstrations of nonpharmacologic pain relief measures such as massage, aromatherapy, music therapy, and meditation. Nursing support for caregivers should encourage personal contributions to the comfort of a loved one during a difficult time. After the patient dies, the caregiver may be consoled by the memory that they were able to assist with the comfort care.

Nurses have a responsibility to develop a realistic plan of care with the patient, family, and primary care provider that honors the patient's wishes and addresses physical and emotional needs of both the dying person and the caregivers. To fulfill that responsibility, nurses need to understand the basic processes of dying and ways of applying the nursing process to the dying process.

End-of-life processes

In all except the sudden death trajectory, there are recognizable changes that occur over time at the end of life. A nurse attending a dying patient can observe the signs of transition toward death. Although each person's death is unique, there are common patterns that the nurse, the family, and other care providers can observe and use to understand what is happening and then to modify wound considerations and other interventions to fit individual needs.

The dying process is a natural slowing down of physical and mental processes. Signs and symptoms may occur days or weeks before death or may be present only hours or minutes before. Often the first signs as a patient nears the end of life are psychologic and spiritual in nature. Expressions of fear about the dying process, fear of abandonment, and fear of the unknown are common. An increased focus on the spiritual aspects of life and a renewed search for meaning are common, as is a withdrawal from family, friends, and caregivers as death approaches [2]. The phenomenon of an awareness of nearing death, in which patients try to communicate a special understanding about dying and often attempt to relate their experiences symbolically or metaphorically, is often observed among those close to death [10].

Signs and symptoms at the end of life include changes in cognition, activity level, oral intake of food and fluids, and changes in bowel and bladder elimination. Each of these areas is briefly discussed below, and ramifications for wound care are then addressed within the nursing process framework.

Mental changes

Mental changes such as confusion, disorientation, and delirium are often observed at EOL. Normal human cognition is dependent on a complex balance of physiologic factors, all of which are generally disrupted as death approaches. Cognitive changes include impairment in the level of consciousness and alteration in the ability to discern detail, accuracy of perception, and memory loss [11]. When mental status changes initially occur, an assessment should be performed to rule out causes that can be remedied to increase comfort. For example, if the mental changes are related to fever from wound infection, antibiotic treatment may be indicated. The possibility that observed changes in mental status are part of the nearing death awareness phenomenon should also be considered.

As the dying process continues, increased drowsiness, more sleeping, and a decreased level of responsiveness to stimuli are often observed. Prolonged periods of inactivity place patients, who are often already debilitated from the terminal disease experience, at much greater risk for tissue damage.

Activity changes

Other activity level changes also accompany end-of-life transitions. Patients may experience more weakness and fatigue than previously. It is not uncommon, however, for a patient to experience a surge of energy a few days before dying. Patients who have been generally lethargic sometimes seem to experience a rally of spirit and energy just before the final active phase of dying. Many patients have a period of increased restlessness, with or without delirium, and some demonstrate what is called terminal agitation or terminal anguish. This condition is characterized by marked restlessness, with moans and crying that do not seem responsive to comfort measures. Sedation of the patient is sometimes used at this point to relieve distress for the family unable to watch their loved one in apparent unrelieved discomfort [11].

Food and fluid intake changes

One of the hallmarks of the dying process is the change that normally occurs in intake of food and fluids. As organ systems shut down, the dying person no longer needs or wants to eat or drink. This decrease in oral intake, like many of the other patterns discussed, may begin to appear weeks or months before death and is usually extremely distressing to family and caregivers [2,11]. In many cultures, food is equated with care, nurturance, spirituality, and life itself. The cessation of feeding, even when the person no longer wants to eat and the physical body no longer requires or is able to process food, is a critical point for both patient and family. The same pattern is true with regard to decreasing and then stopping fluid intake in terminal illness. The swallow reflex often decreases or disappears at the end of life, making oral intake difficult. Fluids given parenterally and nutrition given by tube feeding are not usually appropriate at the end of life. These interventions may help the family feel that they are doing something, but tubes and lines increase discomfort for the dying person, inhibit what little mobility the person may have, lead to uncomfortable bowel and bladder distention, and do nothing to prolong or increase the quality of life.

Elimination changes

Near the end of life changes in bowel elimination such as diarrhea and constipation are common. Urinary incontinence is also frequently observed. The cause and pathophysiology of these symptoms and recommended interventions are beyond the scope of this discussion and are treated extensively elsewhere [12–14]. Decreased food and fluid intake, mobility decline, and changes in muscle and nerve function are all associated with elimination changes. Medications also have side effects for bowel and bladder function. For constipation, prevention is the best treatment, and careful assessment is paramount; for diarrhea and urinary incontinence, the challenges to wound care, particularly wounds in the sacral and perineal areas, are great.

Imminent death

The signs and symptoms of dying vary widely depending on factors such as the patient's health status before illness, age, disease diagnosis, comorbidities, and many other factors. There are, however, signs that are more universal that indicate that death is imminent in a matter of hours or minutes. The onset of these signs is the start of what is called the active dying phase. Decreased urine output, cold and mottled arms and legs, and changes in vital signs are usually noted at this point. Respiratory congestion, including a bubbling sound, is common, and the patient's breathing pattern changes [2,15]. Paramount at this stage of the dying process is attention to patient comfort and relief of distressing symptoms using the least invasive measures possible.

At time of death and after

Signs and symptoms of death include absence of heart beat and respirations, release of stool and urine, unresponsiveness, fixed and dilated pupils, a pale, waxen appearance of skin, and decreasing body temperature. The dying person's eyes usually remain open, and the jaw often drops, opening the mouth. Because breathing is often irregular in the last hours and minutes, with periods of apnea and rapid shallow breaths, the last breath may be quite difficult to identify. Movement of the body postmortem sometimes results in an additional release of air from the lungs and can be mistaken for an additional breath from the patient. Official pronouncement of death is governed by policies in place in various health care organizations and agencies [16].

The Kennedy terminal ulcer [17] is a pressure ulcer that may be detected late in the dying process. It usually occurs on the sacrum and appears pear-shaped with irregular borders. The onset is sudden, and the tissue deterioration progresses quickly. If indicated, treatment for a Kennedy ulcer follows the same guidelines as stage III–IV. However, because this type of wound occurs very close to the time of death, it is often left untreated.

At this delicate time, when the family wants to see their loved one, the nurse should consider changing or covering an existing dressing with the intent to have the patient appear clean and without odor. During these last few minutes, the family needs to feel the patient was well cared for, treated with respect and dignity, and is now at peace.

Nursing process with wounds at end of life

Assessment, diagnosis, planning, intervention, and evaluation guide wound care at the end of life as in all other stages across the lifespan. The nursing process, central to the discipline of nursing, suggests an organized consideration of some of the critical factors in EOL wound care. Nursing process is not linear and sequential as discussed but rather circular and recursive as practiced. Critical thinking on the part of the professional nurse is essential to the nursing process and to excellent patient care. Priorities for EOL wound care using the classic Leavell and Clark [18] framework include primary prevention (avoidance of wounds), secondary prevention (early identification and treatment), and tertiary prevention (care, healing, or avoidance of additional damage, pain, and suffering).

Assessment

Comprehensive assessment is the foundation for application of the nursing process at end of life. Systematic physical, psychologic, social, and spiritual assessments are indicated as well as specific consideration of actual or potential areas of loss of skin integrity. Listed below are some areas on which to focus assessment with regard to EOL wounds.

Overall condition

- What are the clinical signs and symptoms of disease progression, risk factors, comorbidities, and progression of dying? What is the patient's most likely death trajectory?
- What is the patient's Karnofsky Performance Status score? A score of 50% or less indicates significant diminished functional status and increased risk for skin breakdown [19].
- How does the patient rate on the Braden Risk Assessment Scale? Scores range from 4 to 23, with lower scores indicating higher risk for skin breakdown [20,21].
- Is the patient having urinary or fecal incontinence? Is incontinence contributing to skin breakdown or complicating wound care?

- What is the patient's mental state? Can the patient direct or participate in wound care at this time? If restless or confused, is the patient at higher risk for injury?
- What is the patient's current fluid and nutritional intake? How are appetite and desire for food and fluids? Are there lesions in the mouth or throat that affect intake and comfort?

General integument

- Does a thorough head-to-toe observation of the patient's skin reveal any areas of loss or threatened loss of integrity?
- Pay special attention to areas over bony prominences, surgical sites, prior intravenous and central line insertion sites, radiation sites, and any other areas that are subject to pressure, friction, or other mechanical, chemical, or thermal damage.

Specific wounds

- How are the wound characteristics described using the acronym CLOSED: Color, Location, Odor, Size, Exudate, and Depth.
- What is the stage of each ulcer using National Pressure Ulcer Advisory Panel definitions [15]?
- How long has the patient had the wound?
- What treatments or dressings have been applied? By whom? With what effect?

Pain and other symptom discomfort

- What is the patient's current pain rating on numerical or visual analog scales of 0 to 10 [22,23]?
- What is the patient's description of pain? What are the observed signs of pain?
- Keep in mind that pain experience and pain reporting occur within cultural, spiritual, and religious contexts. The meaning of pain and suffering at the end of life are highly variable and influence patient and family acceptance and responses to pain interventions.
- Does treatment of existing ulcers or other wounds exacerbate or alleviate patient pain?

Diagnosis and planning

When considering nursing diagnosis in the terminal phase, the goals of the patient and family are most important. Nursing diagnoses for terminally ill patients are as widely varied as for patients at any other stage of life. However, the focus usually turns away from diagnoses that suggest activities for a cure or a return to function. The focus now is on those problems, needs, and strengths that the patient and family identify as important for life closure and a "good death." Diagnoses and intervention plans that address needs for care, comfort, and dignity (as defined by the dying patient and loved ones) are most commonly appropriate. Some considerations in this part of the nursing process include

- Involving the patient in care planning to the extent feasible and desired by the patient and family
- Identifying the patient and family goals for a "good death"
- Aligning proposed wound care plans with patient and family goals, for example,

    If control of pain is a central goal, how do wound treatment or wound prevention measures affect patient pain?
    If maximum mobility for as long as possible is a central goal, how does the wound plan accommodate or impede movement?
    If visitation by friends and family is a central goal, how do wound coverings and odor control plans fit with patient and family expectations?

- Identifying strengths and assets that can be drawn on to help meet the care goals, such as

    How much time is the caregiver present? Who else is available to help?
    To what degree are the caregivers capable of assisting with basic patient needs?
    Is the caregiver willing to perform wound care?

Interventions

Prevention measures

Clearly, the best intervention for wounds is prevention. If the patient has not yet developed wounds, or to avoid development of additional wounds, common interventions to maintain skin integrity include

- Providing therapeutic and comfortable support surfaces

    When suggesting a pressure reduction overlay or mattress for the patient's bed, also evaluate the need for a cushion for a favorite chair or recliner. Often a chair is the favorite place for the patient to spend the most time relaxing or even sleeping. Choose cushions and overlays based on comfort for the patient, ease of use (size, washable material, etc.), and cost.

- Avoiding the use of donut-shaped cushions because these cause increased pressure around the edges and may lead to preventable skin breakdown
- Placing a small pillow just under the leg, proximal to the heels, to suspend the heels enough to prevent breakdown for a patient in bed

Heels are at high risk for breakdown among immobile patients. Remember that knee and ankle joints also need to be supported.

- Individualizing the bathing schedule based on patient needs

  Use a gentle cleanser, soft cloths, tepid water, and pat the skin dry. Do not rub or massage.

- Applying lotion without perfume

  Perfume may act as a skin irritant and the scent may be offensive to the patient.

- Keeping the patient's nails short to avoid injury or skin tearing

  The caregiver's nails should also be kept short.

- Avoiding tight fitting clothing and seams that could cause unnecessary pressure and discomfort
- Cleaning the patient quickly after incontinent episodes

  Try to avoid use of diapers. If the situation requires diapers, use products that wick the moisture away from the skin, and change the diapers when soiled [5].

Dressing wounds

The most universal intervention for wounds is the application of dressings. General criteria for appropriate dressings are (1) protection of the wound, (2) decrease in pain and discomfort, (3) provision of an environment for healing, and (4) the ability for the dressing to remain intact for 3 to 7 days. For many people in the final days and weeks of life, criteria 2 and 4 take precedence. Certainly, wound care interventions should not further harm the patient by increasing wound size or causing infection if such can be avoided. Wound healing is not a primary goal when the patient is near death. Dressings that alleviate pain and avoid unnecessary discomfort and dressings that remain intact for longer periods of time are most desirable. Specific dressing considerations for EOL wounds include

- Matching the wound treatment options to the patient's overall condition, level of pain, wound assessment, ease of use, wear time, cost-effectiveness, and level of caregiver ability
- Not using dressings that will adhere to the wound bed, thereby causing unnecessary pain and discomfort (ie, avoid "wet-to-dry" dressings)
- If moderate to heavy exudates are present, choosing a dressing that will minimize the frequency of dressing changes while absorbing the drainage, protecting the skin around the wound, and controlling odor [5]

Turn and position

Regular turning and positioning of patients to prevent pressure ulcers is taught as essential nursing care for all patients with compromised mobility. When the patient is terminally ill, however, this intervention needs to be carefully, critically, and continuously evaluated. Although the patient is in the early phases of dying, repositioning for comfort and relief from prolonged pressure may be appropriate. Interventions during this early period include

- Fostering activity that is desired and tolerated by the patient

  Coordinate activity with the administration of pain medication so that the activity is performed when the patient is most comfortable.

- Considering an over-bed trapeze to help the patient move with less discomfort and maintain maximum independence for as long as possible
- Teaching the patient and caregiver how to safely transfer between surfaces

  Proper transfer technique will decrease potential for skin breakdown and will reduce caregiver risk for injury.

- Keeping bed linen clean and wrinkle-free

  Use a drawsheet to lift the patient when repositioning to decrease skin and tissue damage from friction.

When death becomes imminent, turning and repositioning cause undue suffering and should be discontinued. Minimizing the amount of manipulation and movement the patient must endure contributes to maximum comfort. In the active dying phase, the patient no longer needs a change of position, bed linen, or dressings, and the pursuit of these things detracts from peace and dignity at the time of death.

Nutritional support

Nurses routinely teach patients and families that wounds need proper nutrition to heal. At the end of life, when physical healing is no longer a goal, nutrition and hydration needs change. The decreased need for nourishment and hydration is part of the dying process. Forcing food or fluid intake at the end of life only serves to make the dying person less comfortable and to worsen other symptoms. Some interventions to consider with regard to intake include

- Honoring the patient's food and fluid preferences and do not force intake

  Offer frequent small feedings of favorite foods.

- Minimizing food odors if this is a problem for the patient

  Sometimes cold foods are better tolerated and less offensive.

- Trying various nutritional supplements in small amounts to see if there is one the patient enjoys and can tolerate during the early phases of the terminal illness
- Offering fluids including ice chips or popsicles during early and middle phases
- Assisting with oral care to increase comfort and hygiene especially in active dying phase
- Teaching the family about the normal process of food and fluid withdrawal at EOL

Food and drink are generally considered to be central components of humanity across cultural groups, and the declining interest and ability to maintain food intake are often very distressing to family members.

Evaluation

The final step in the nursing process brings the nurse, patient, and family back to the beginning. Evaluation includes ongoing assessment of the patient and family status and the responses to care. Initially, the nurse should inspect the skin at least daily for redness, discoloration, and blisters. More frequent inspection is necessary as the patient's condition deteriorates as death draws near. Incorporating skin evaluation with necessary care such as bathing can minimize discomfort. Continuous evaluation of the patient and family goals along with assessment of goal achievement and refining of interventions increases the chance that terminal care will be appropriate.

Summary

Nurses are in a unique and privileged position with regard to both end-of-life care and wound care. Expert wound care can greatly contribute to the relief of physiologic stress on the human organism and psychosocial and physical distress at the end of life. Using what is known from both domains, nurses apply critical thinking to assist patients, families, and other caregivers in maintaining the maximum possible integrity of the physical body of the dying person. The manner in which nurses approach wound care with dying patients and the ability to preserve patient dignity and family respect while doing necessary palliative interventions also can serve the healing of emotional wounds in the dying process.

References

[1] Kausler DH, Kausler BC. The graying of America: an encyclopedia of aging, health, mind, and behavior [electronic version]. Available at: http://www.press.uillinois.edu/s01/kausler.html. Accessed October 23, 2004.

[2] End-of-Life Nursing Education Consortium (ELNEC). Training program: faculty guide. Washington (DC): American Association of Colleges of Nursing and City of Hope National Medical Center; 2002.

[3] Galvin J. An audit of pressure ulcer incidence in a palliative care setting. Int J Palliat Nurs 2002;8(5):214, 216, 218–21.

[4] Hanson D, Langemo D, Olson B, et al. The prevalence and incidence of pressure ulcers in the hospice setting : analysis of two methodologies. Am J Hosp Palliat Care 1991;8(5):18–22.

[5] Bryant R, editor. Acute and chronic wounds: nursing management. St. Louis (MO): Mosby; 2000.

[6] Miller C. Nursing aspects of symptoms management. In: Doyle D, Hanks G, MacDonald N, editors. Oxford textbook of palliative medicine. 2nd edition. New York: Oxford University Press; 1998. p. 642–56.

[7] Glaser BG, Strauss AL. Time for dying. Chicago: Aldine Press; 1968.

[8] National Hospice and Palliative Care Organization (NHPCO) Web site. (2004). An explanation of palliative care. Available at: http://www.nhpco.org/i4a/pages/index.cfm. pageid = 3657. Accessed March 8, 2004.

[9] US Department of Health and Human Sevices. Medicare hospice benefits. 2000. Baltimore (MD): US Department of Health and Human Services; Publication No. CMS 02154. July 2003. Available at: http://www.medicare.gov/publications/pubs/pdf/02154.pdf. Accessed October 23, 2004.

[10] Callahan M, Kelley P, editors. Final gifts: understanding the special awareness, needs, and communications of the dying. New York: Bantam; 1997.

[11] Kuebler KK, English N, Heidrich DE. Delirium, confusion, agitation, and restlessness. In: Ferrell BR, Coyle N, editors. Textbook of palliative nursing. New York: Oxford University Press; 2001. p. 290–308.

[12] Kuebler KK, Berry PH, Heidrich DE, editors. End-of-life care: clinical practice guidelines. Philadelphia: Saunders; 2002.

[13] Economou DC. Bowel management: Constipation, diarrhea, obstruction, and ascites. In: Ferrell BR, Coyle N, editors. Textbook of palliative nursing. New York: Oxford University Press; 2001. p. 139–55.

[14] Matzo ML, Sherman DW, editors. Palliative care nursing: quality care to the end of life. New York: Springer; 2001.

[15] Berry P, Griffie J. Planning for the actual death. In: Ferrell BR, Coyle N, editors. Textbook of palliative nursing. New York: Oxford University Press; 2001. p. 392–6.

[16] Kemp C. Terminal illness: a guide to nursing care. 2nd edition. Philadelphia: Lippincott; 1999.

[17] Kennedy KL. The prevalence of pressure ulcers in an intermediate care facility. Decubitus 1989;2(2):44–5.

[18] Leavell HR, Clark EG. Preventive medicine for the doctor in his community. New York: McGraw-Hill; 1958.

[19] Osaba D, MacDonald N. Disease-modifying management. In: Doyle D, Hanks G, MacDonald N, editors. Oxford textbook of palliative medicine. 2nd edition. New York: Oxford University Press; 1998. p. 255–6.

[20] Bergstrom N, Braden B, Laguzza A, et al. The Braden Scale for predicting pressure sores at risk. Nurs Res 1987;36(4):205–10.

[21] Agency for Health Care Policy and Research (AHCPR). Pressure ulcers in adults: prediction and prevention. Rockville (MD): U.S. Department of Health and Human Services, Public Health Service, AHPCR; 1992. AHCPR Publication #92-0047. http://www.ncbi.nlm.nih.gov/books/bv.fcgi?rid = hstat2.chapter.4409. Accessed October 23, 2004.

[22] Dalton JA, MacNaull F. A call for standardizing the clinical rating of pain intensity using a 0–10 rating scale. Cancer Nurs 1998;21:46–9.

[23] Gift AG. Visual analogue scales: measurement of subjective phenomena. Nurs Res 1989; 38(5):286–8.

ELSEVIER
SAUNDERS

Nurs Clin N Am 40 (2005) 295–323

NURSING
CLINICS
OF NORTH AMERICA

Wound Care Issues in the Patient with Cancer

Mary A. Gerlach, MSN, APRN-BC, CWOCN

Division of Nursing, St. Joseph's Mercy of Macomb Hospital, 15855 Nineteen Mile Road, Clinton Township, MI 48038, USA

Individuals with cancer often suffer from acute or chronic wounds [1,2] that are caused by the disease or the effects of cancer treatment; and these wounds present many challenges for the patient, family, and health care team [1]. In addition to dealing with the diagnosis of cancer, the presence of a wound serves as a persistent reminder of the disease and treatment [3]. Disruption of the skin by cancer may result in open wounds that bleed, become infected, are malodorous, and cause pain [1,4,5]. Injuries resulting from cancer treatment may range from superficial areas of skin loss to extensive areas of tissue necrosis, resulting in permanent damage and disfigurement [1,3,5]. According to Magnan [6], an individual's psychological response to a wound may be closely related to the mechanism of wounding. This rationale offers insight into why cancer patients with wounds may have difficulty with symptom management, disturbances of body image, decreased feelings of self-worth, and alterations in their quality of life [1,7]. Nursing management of the cancer patient with a wound requires an understanding of the normal phases of wound healing, basic wound care principles, and the alterations that may accompany the disease process [1,4]. By using this knowledge base, nurses can minimize the negative impact of the wound and optimize the quality of life for the patient.

Normal wound healing

Skin injury initiates a cascade of four phases of wound healing: hemostasis, the inflammatory phases, the proliferative phase, and the maturation phase, which aids in wound closure [4,8,9]. Within each phase of

E-mail address: gerlachm@trinity-health.org

0029-6465/05/$ - see front matter © 2005 Elsevier Inc. All rights reserved.
doi:10.1016/j.cnur.2004.09.008

wound healing, critical cellular elements are attracted to the wound to aid healing [9]. These elements, such as platelets, fibroblasts, macrophages, and endothelial cells, among others, must be present in adequate supply for the phases of healing to progress sequentially [9]. Initially after injury, platelets are produced and cause hemostasis and clot formation [9]. Neutrophils and macrophages are then released to mount an acute inflammatory response. Fibroblasts are produced in the proliferative phase to aid formation of granulation tissue, wound contraction, and scar formation, or re-epithelialization [9]. In the maturation phase, scar tissue undergoes remodeling to increase the tensile strength of the wounded area [9].

Impaired wound healing and cancer

The presence of cancer and the effects of cancer therapy cause alterations in normal wound healing [4,10]. Malnutrition is the comorbid condition most commonly found in cancer patients. Nutritional compromise is associated with delayed skin repair and poor wound healing [1,4]. Patients undergoing chemotherapy or radiation therapy are at risk for protein-calorie malnutrition [1,4]. Chemotherapy causes neutropenia and thrombocytopenia, which decreases the availability of inflammatory cells such as neutrophils and platelets for skin repair [1,4]. These deficits render a patient more susceptible to infection and prolong the inflammatory phase of wound healing by impairing macrophage function [1,4]. Because the principal role of the neutrophil is phagocytosis, the patient's primary defense against infection is reduced [4]. Radiation therapy disrupts mitotic reproduction in the basal membrane, which can lead to thinning of the epidermis and even fibrosis of the dermis [1,11].

Relationship between cancer and wounds and malignancies that present as wounds

Cancer may initially present as a wound, but wounds may also develop cancer [1,2,3]. Additionally, injury may also result from chemotherapy extravasation and from the acute and delayed effects of radiation therapy [1,4]. The most common malignancies that may present as wounds include untreated basal cell carcinoma, squamous cell carcinoma, and melanoma (which can be a manifestation of metastatic or primary disease) [3,12]. A classic example of this phenomenon is a "rodent ulcer," which denotes a basal cell carcinoma that outgrows its blood supply, erodes, and subsequently ulcerates [3]. The presentation of these lesions varies and may be mistaken for a sore that will not heal or is otherwise benign [3]. Because only 3% of malignancies present initially as ulcers, and malignant transformations are even less common, the diagnosis is often delayed [3,13].

Atypical wounds associated with cancer

Certain atypical wounds also may occur simultaneously with cancer [3]. This presentation is often seen with inflammatory ulcers such as pyoderma gangrenosum (PG) and vasculitis [3,12]. Pyoderma gangrenosum is an inflammatory process of unknown causes characterized by one or more painful, chronic necrotizing ulcers with violaceous undermined borders [12]. Pyoderma gangrenosum is associated with several other conditions, including cancer and inflammatory bowel disease in up to 75% of patients [12]. Vasculitis is defined as inflammation and necrosis of the blood vessels that may affect any organ or system, including the skin, and may result in end-organ damage [12]. Vasculitis represents a reaction pattern that may be caused by certain triggers such as infections, medications, connective tissue diseases, and cancer [12]. The clinical presentation of vasculitis depends on the size of the underlying vessels that are affected. Presentation can vary from reticulated erythema to widespread purpura, necrosis, and ulceration [12].

Cancer treatment that may result in wounds

Certain cancer treatments have been linked with the development of wounds [3]. The chemotherapeutic agent hydroxyurea has been linked to the development of leg ulcers [3]. The use of ionizing radiation for treatment of tumors may result in the development of chronic, nonhealing ulcers [3,12].

Cancer development in chronic wounds

Cancer may also develop within a chronic wound. A chronic wound that undergoes malignant transformation is referred to as Marjolin's ulcer [3,12]. Marjolin's ulcer is a rare (2% of chronic wounds) and often aggressive cutaneous malignancy that arises in previously traumatized or chronically inflamed skin [3,12]. This phenomenon may also occur in burns, chronic pressure ulcers, diabetes, sinus tracts, chronic osteomyelitis, vaccination sites, irradiated skin, and venous ulcers [3,12]. With chronic venous ulcers, the risk of developing a malignancy is 21% [3]. Marjolin's ulcers typically affect 40- to 70-year-old men who have had osteomyelitis and chronic wounds of the lower extremities for a period of 20 to 50 years; however these ulcers have been reported to appear as early as 18 months [3]. Squamous cell carcinoma is the type of neoplasm most commonly associated with Marjolin's ulcers [3].

Causes of cancer in chronic wounds

The precise mechanism by which malignancy develops in wounds is not known but is thought to be an example of wound healing gone awry [3,12]. Several different complex mechanisms have been proposed to explain this occurrence [3,12]. Chronic irritation and infection have been cited as major factors that may lead to the development of a malignant clone in a wound and the subsequent development of cancer [3,12].

Wound biopsy

Chronic wounds will not heal in the presence of tumor cells [3,12]. Controversy about the proper time to obtain a biopsy exists among experts [3]. Because only 2% of chronic wounds undergoes malignant transformation, some authors recommend performing a biopsy only on suspicious wounds [3,12]. Any ulcer that appears abnormal, for example, with thick and rolled edges, should undergo biopsy for a definitive diagnosis [12]. The treatment of biopsy-confirmed cancers depends on the type and extent of the wound [3,14].

Malignant cutaneous wounds

Cutaneous metastatic skin lesions are extensions of a tumor in the skin [2,5,8]. Malignant cutaneous wounds (MCWs) are defined as breaks in epidermal integrity caused by malignant cell infiltration [2,5,7]. These wounds represent primary or metastatic malignant skin lesions that are different in location and progression from traditionally encountered wounds [1,2,5,7]. Cutaneous metastasis usually occurs through the lymphatics, bloodstream, or directly from a primary lesion [3]. Cutaneous metastasis may also develop along a suture line, following surgery for a primary tumor, from recurrence of cancer, or through mechanical implantation via a diagnostic or operative procedure [3,14].

MCWs may present as the initial sign of cancer or as a result of metastasis late in the course of the disease [3,15]. MCWs are usually the result of metastasis rather than a primary skin lesion [3]. In most cases, the presence of a tumor in the skin occurs concurrently with sites of metastatic disease [1]. Generally, cutaneous metastases are associated with end-stage disease, and the expected survival is often less than 1 year [1,2,8]. The incidence of MCWs is difficult to establish, but has been reported in up to 9% of patients with cancer [2,16]. The incidence of MCWs positively correlates with incidence rates for primary cancer sites [2]. After melanoma, malignant skin lesions occur most frequently among women with breast cancer (19% to 50%) and with bronchogenic carcinoma (3% to 8%) [7,15]. Malignant skin lesions may also occur with head and neck, stomach, kidney, uterine, ovarian, colon, bladder cancers, and lymphoma [2,8].

Characteristics of malignant cutaneous wounds

Most metastatic skin lesions occur on the anterior trunk but may be found on any part of the body [3,7]. MCWs present variously as small, firm, flesh-colored nodules just under the surface of the skin to large, fungating lesions [2,7,15]. These lesions may occur individually or in groups and may be pink, red, violet, or brown [2,7,15]. Patients may be asymptomatic or may experience pruritus, pain, stinging, or macular rash, and thickening and hardening of the skin [15]. Presenting symptoms have little to do with the size of the lesion [15].

The British Columbia Cancer Agency (2001) defines an ulcerating malignant skin lesion as a cancerous lesion involving the skin that is open and draining [16]. Malignant cells that penetrate the surrounding lymph and blood circulation lead to capillary enlargement and possible rupture, causing the alterations seen with MCWs [2,7,16]. Because of ischemia or metabolite toxicity or a combination of these factors, this process can lead to the formation of a necrotic core [2,7,16]. The necrotic core quickly leads to the characteristic skin breakdown of MCWs [2,5]. MCWs are frequently exudative, hemorrhagic, and odorous [6,16]. These signs are directly related to alterations in wound healing secondary to cancer [1,2]. Wounds caused by tumors lack the ability to contract [1,2,15]; therefore, as healing occurs, a larger deficit occurs compared with normal wound healing [2,15]. The result of these alterations is a wound that drains and may never fully close and that is subject to opportunistic infection [1,2].

Assessment of malignant cutaneous wounds

Care of a patient with MCWs begins with knowledge of the specific type of cancer, extent of disease, and goals of care [2]. Unlike other wounds, symptom control is the primary focus of management rather than healing [2,7,15,16]. These wounds usually have a poor outcome, and it is generally accepted that resolution is not the primary goal of care, particularly in the absence of effective therapy [2,7]. However, surgery, chemotherapy, or radiotherapy, when used to treat the underlying disease, may assist in controlling a MCW [2,16,17].

Treatment options for malignant cutaneous wounds

External beam radiation therapy may be an option for the control of local metastases [15]. Radiation destroys tumor cells, thereby reducing the mass of a lesion, which can lead to decreased exudate and pain [1,15]. Chemotherapy may be used to relieve tumor symptoms and is administered with the consideration of previous therapy [15]. Surgery may be used to excise or debulk the tumor mass but may have a limited role if the mass extends into and involves other surrounding structures [15].

Research into new therapies for breast cancer, including cutaneous metastatic lesions, promises more effective treatment for these often resistant sites [15]. Agents currently undergoing clinical trials include photodynamic therapy using porfimer sodium (PhotoFrin, Axcan Pharma, Inc., Birmingham, AL), miltefosine (Miltex, Asta Medica, Frankfort, Germany), and antiangiogenesis agents [15].

When treatments are ineffective, palliative wound management is necessary [7]. Little research has been conducted regarding MCWs [2,15,16]. Existing nursing and medical literature describes exploratory management approaches, symptom management, and a framework for assessment and staging of MCWs [2]. A classic report by Foltz [2], in 1980, describes six key areas for local care of MCWs, including cleansing, debridement, reduction of superficial bacterial flora, control of bleeding, reduction of odor, and dressings. Presently, no universal guidelines exist to objectively describe a MCW, its size, changes over time, or the best method of treatment [2,15,16].

Care of the patient with an MCW should be directed toward alleviation of symptoms that are most concerning to the patient [2,5,15]. The patient's emotional and social adjustment to the wound should be incorporated, as well as identifying support systems and the individual who will assist the patient with wound care [5].

Assessment of an MCW should include the same criteria used with other wounds, including location, appearance, size, amount and character of drainage, odor, presence of infection, surrounding skin integrity, percentage of devitalized tissue in the wound bed, and effects of treatment such as radiation or chemotherapy [2,18]. Wound descriptions should be documented in a concise and systematic manner to increase reliability with ongoing assessments [2]. The Malignant Cutaneous Wound Staging study (1997) [2] demonstrated the value of using wound photographs to document changes over time.

Local wound management

If the overlying skin is intact, no wound management is required other than protection [15]. The patient should be taught strategies for wound protection, including using a protective cover and wearing loose clothing to prevent friction [15]. Local care should address basic wound care principles, including cleansing and debridement to decrease bacterial levels and risk of infection; maintaining a moist wound environment to reduce trauma and bleeding and aid granulation and re-epithelialization where possible; managing odor and exudate; selecting the type of dressing according to individual wound needs; and enhancing comfort and body image [5,7,15,17]. Wound products should prevent maceration and irritation, absorb drainage, and reduce the risk of skin stripping with dressing changes [5,16,17].

Odor is a distressing problem for patients, families, and members of the health care team. Odor may be caused by the presence of necrotic tissue, colonization or infection, and saturated dressings [6,16,17]. The hypoxic environment of an MCW promotes bacterial proliferation, which establishes a destructive, prolonged inflammatory cycle in wound healing [2,19]. Necrotic tissue may be heavily colonized with anaerobic bacteria, which form volatile fatty acid end products that cause foul wound odors [2,5]. Reduction of the necrosis and infection will alleviate much of the odor [2]. Interventions to reduce odor include changing dressings before they become saturated, wound cleansing, charcoal-impregnated dressings; and treatment of infection, debridement, and the use of metronidazole [5,7]. Lawrence et al [20] studied the odor-reducing capabilities of five different dressings containing active charcoal [5,17]. All of the dressings effectively reduced odor, but the bacterial content of wound drainage was unchanged, and the ability to absorb drainage varied [5,17]. Room deodorizers, yogurt, and buttermilk have demonstrated only minimal success in reducing odor [16].

Several studies [21] have demonstrated the effectiveness of metronidazole in reducing or eliminating odor in malodorous wounds. Metronidazole is bactericidal and trichomonacidal and reduces odor by reducing the number of bacteria in the wound [21]. Both topical metronidazole (Metro Gel topical gel, 0.75%) and oral metronidazole have demonstrated odor reduction in MCWs [11]. Although not an approved use for metronidazole, some clinicians report [7,11] success in applying dressings that have been soaked in a solution of normal saline combined with crushed metronidazole tablets.

Wound cleansing removes bacteria and necrotic debris from a wound [5,17]. The long-term goal of wound care with MCWs, especially if the patient is receiving chemotherapy, is to minimize the bacterial burden in the wound [15]. Because MCWs are heavily colonized with anaerobic bacteria, the goal is to prevent the spread of bacteria to the surrounding or underlying tissue and to prevent systemic infection or sepsis [15]. Wound infection is usually diagnosed through clinical signs such as cellulitis, fever, and leuko-cytosis [15]. These signs warrant systemic antibiotic therapy [15]. Classic signs of infection may not be present in chronic wounds or in a patient who is immunosuppressed [22]. Pain may be the only sign of wound infection in these patients [15].

MCWs should be cleansed by gentle irrigation rather than swabbing [7,18]. Options for wound cleansing solutions may include normal saline or a noncytoxic surfactant cleanser [5,7,17]. In wounds with heavy exudates or adherent material, a commercial wound cleanser containing surfactants helps to remove wound contaminants [5,17]. The cleansing method should provide enough pressure to remove debris yet not cause trauma to the wound bed [5,17]. This is especially critical with MCWs because excessive irrigation pressure can aggravate bleeding in an already friable wound

[7,17]. The optimal pressure for wound cleansing is between 4 and 15 psi [23]. The use of a 250-mL bottle of normal saline solution with an attached irrigation cap (Baxter, Deerfield, IL) is an effective yet safe way (at a pressure of 5 psi) to cleanse MCWs [7]. Alternatively, a daily shower can also accomplish this goal [7]. Antiseptics should not be used for wound cleansing because they are cytotoxic, nonselective, and may cause trauma to the wound bed [19]. To date, no scientifically valid clinical studies have documented the antibacterial benefits of using antiseptics in chronic wounds [19].

Debridement removes necrotic tissue, which is a medium for bacterial colonization and odor [5,7]. Simply cleansing a wound may debride or remove some necrotic tissue [5]. The application of a hydrogel dressing is a gentle method to facilitate autolytic debridement [5,17]. A temporary increase in wound odor and drainage may occur with hydrogel debridement [5,17]. Enzymatic debridement involves the use of natural proteases to facilitate removal of necrotic debris while sparing normal tissue [5,11]. For wounds with wet necrotic tissue, polysaccharide or starch copolymer beads are effective for debridement [5]. Surgical debridement is rarely used with MCWs [11]. Mechanical debridement using wet-to-dry dressings is not recommended because of the associated pain and bleeding that may occur in MCWs [11,17].

Spontaneous or intermittent bleeding can occur in MCWs because of capillary erosion and the absence of platelets within the tumor stroma [5,7]. Bleeding can be anxiety provoking as well as life threatening [5]. A variety of agents can be used to control local bleeding, including nonadherent dressings, local pressure applied for 10 to 15 minutes, hemostatic agents such as silver nitrate sticks, oxidized cellulose dressings (Gelfoam), and the application of topical adrenaline 1:1000 (1mg/1mL) for emergent situations [11]. Wound ischemia may occur with the use of adrenaline [11]. For controlling light bleeding, gentle cleansing and alginate dressings may be effective [11].

The skin surrounding an MCW is vulnerable to epidermal skin stripping, maceration, and infection [5,15]. Prevention measures include the use of skin barriers such as liquid film barriers, skin barrier wafers, cream, or ointment, and containment of wound drainage with an ostomy or wound pouch [5,15]. Additional measures include regular dressing changes to prevent pooling or "strike through" of drainage, use of absorbent dressings, and absorbent underpads used as dressings [5,11].

Dressings selected for MCWs should be absorbent, prevent adherence, and maintain a moist wound environment [5]. Appropriate dressings include gauze impregnated with hydrogel or petrolatum, foam dressings, and alginates [17]. The frequency of dressing change depends on the volume of exudates produced and the amount of necrotic tissues present, and the patient's hydration status and activity level [5]. Open wounds with little exudate can be packed with dry gauze and covered with a nonadherent dressing [15]. If dressings adhere to the wound bed, the use of petroleum-impregnated gauze will protect the wound bed [15,17]. Petrolatum dressings should be used cautiously in patients undergoing radiation therapy because residual petroleum can potentiate the bolus effect of radiation [17]. Before radiation, these dressings should be removed, and petrolatum should be cleansed from the wound [17].

The use of tape should be avoided to secure dressings [7,15]. Options to secure dressings to the chest wall include mesh panties with the crotch cut out, a soft sleep bra with hooks in the front, or a loose fitting tube top [5,7]. For other body locations, the use of roller gauze, stretch tubular stockinet, and Exu-Dry (Smith & Nephew) wound dressings and garments may be options. If tape cannot be avoided, the use of nontraumatic, microporous tape is recommended, along with the application of a liquid copolymer film to the skin before tape is applied [5,7].

Pruritus and pain are common subjective symptoms in patients with MCWs. Medications such as diphenhydramine or hydroxyzine may be effective for pruritus [15]. Itching is sometimes relieved with the liberal use of skin lotions or creams [15]. Pain at MCWs is the result of multiple factors [15]. A key source of MCW pain is the trauma associated with dressing changes [15,17]. The use of occlusive dressings may help to relieve pain until some degree of healing takes place [15]. Table 1 presents a chart describing local care of MCWs.

Nurses can also play a role in addressing the psychosocial concerns that arise from the devastation of MCWs [15–17]. Issues such as end-of-life concerns must be addressed by patients, families, and significant others [15–17]. Other needs, including changes in body image, wound odor, drainage, and sexuality, can become issues for individuals and their partners [15]. Counseling both parties, alone and together, may help them to resolve these issues and encourage intimacy [15].

Chemotherapy extravasation in wounds

Extravasation is a severe complication of chemotherapy [24]. When a chemotherapeutic agent leaks into the surrounding tissues, a reaction that varies from skin irritation to necrosis may occur [25]. According to the Intravenous Nurses Society, extravasation is defined as the inadvertent administration of a vesicant solution into surrounding tissue; and infiltration is the advertent administration of a nonvesicant solution into the surrounding tissue [11]. A vesicant is any agent that has the potential to cause blistering or tissue necrosis and may result in severe and long-term tissue damage. An irritant is any agent that causes inflammation but does not cause necrosis, in which symptoms are self-limiting and do not cause long-term sequelae [25]. The incidence of extravasation is unknown because actual injuries are sporadic and underreported, and the terms extravasation and infiltration are frequently interchanged in the literature [26]. The

Table 1
Local care of malignant cutaneous wounds

Nontraumatic dressing changes
  Contact layer
  Gauzes, nonadherent or coated
  Foam
  Protective barrier films (liquid co-polymer skin sealants, eg Skin Prep, NoSting)
  Nontraumatic tapes
Control of bleeding
  Hemostatic agents
  Nonadherent gauze
  Alginates
  Silver nitrate sticks
  Gentle dressing removal
Periwound skin management
  Gentle removal of tape
  Nontraumatic tapes
  Skin sealants (alcohol-free)
  Barrier ointment or cream
  Pectin barrier wafer
Wound Cleansing
  Normal saline
  Noncytotoxic surfactant cleaner
  Showering
Deodorizers
  Charcoal dressings
  Metronidazole (topical or systemic)
Debridement
  Dry, hard, necrotic tissue (hydrogel, enzymatic debriders)
  Wet sloughy tissue (polysaccharide beads, starch, copolymer dressing)
Reduction in wound bioburden
  Cleanse with normal saline or non-surfactant cleaners
  Metronidazole
  Antimicrobial dressings
    Cadexomer iodine
    Silver
    Polyhexamethylene
  Absorptive dressings
  Sodium-impregnated gauze
Exudate Management
  Calcium alginate dressings
  Polysaccharide beads
  Ostomy or wound drainage pouch
  Absorbent pads
  Adult diapers
Attachment Devices (avoid tape)
  Tube top
  Tubular stretch gauze
  Roller gauze
  Stretch net panties with crotch cut out
  Exu-dry
    Wound dressings
    Garments
  Cotton tee shirt

Adapted from Goldberg MT, McGinn-Byer P. Interventions for the fungating wound. In: Bryant RA, editor. Acute and chronic wounds nursing management. 2nd edition. St. Louis MO; Mosby; 2000. p. 376; with permission.

incidence of extravasation is estimated to be between 0.1% and 6% [24–27,29].

Extravasation may occur with any type of peripheral or central vascular access device, including ports [26–29]. Unlike peripheral extravasations, early symptoms of central vascular access device extravasations may be more difficult to detect [26–29]. Tissue damage from port extravasations may be severe and necessitate extensive reconstructive surgery, including simple mastectomy [27–29]. It is estimated that between 0.3% and 4.7% of patients with ports experience extravasations [28]. Schulmeister [28] has noted a dramatic rise in the number of malpractice claims prompted by port extravasations compared with those from peripheral vein extravasations, probably related to the increased use of implanted ports and the severity of harm experienced by these patients. Table 2 lists causes and risk factors for extravasation.

Mechanisms responsible for tissue damage in extravasation

The severity of tissue damage depends on the vesicant potential of the drug, the quantity of drug extravasated, location of the infusion site, tissue response, host factors, and the duration of the process of extravasation [25–27,29]. Tissue damage from vesicant drugs occurs secondarily to one of several mechanisms, including osmotic and pH differences, ischemia, compression, and direct cellular toxicity [25–27,29]. The primary mechanism responsible for tissue damage from vesicant chemotherapy occurs as a result of the ability of the drug to bind with critical cellular structures such as DNA and microtubules [25].

Table 2
Causes and risk factors for extravasation

Causes of extravasation	Risk factors for peripheral extravasation
Backflow secondary to fibrin sheath or thrombosis in CVC	Small, fragile veins
Dislodgment of needle from port	Superior vena cava syndrome
Catheter damage, breakage, or separation of a vascular access device	Peripheral neuropathy
Displacement or migration of the catheter from the vein	Use of medications that produce somnolence, altered mental status, excessive movement, vomiting, coughing
	Veinipuncture technique
	Drug administration technique
	Site of venous access

From Brown KA, Esper P, Kelleher LO, et al, editors. Chemotherapy and biotherapy guidelines and recommendations for practice. Philadelphia: Oncology Nursing Society; 2001. p. 59–63; with permission.

Complications of extravasation

Small extravasations usually do not result in serious problems, and most resolve spontaneously, especially if only a small amount of the drug is infiltrated (less than 0.5 mL) [27]. In severe cases of extravasation (5–7 mL), necrosis, eschar formation, and ulceration with damage of underlying tissues may occur [27]. Three major complications that may result from vesicant extravasation include tissue necrosis and ulceration, compartment syndrome, and reflex sympathetic dystrophy syndrome or chronic pain syndrome [27]. Only one third of extravasations give rise to ulceration [1,27]. Ulceration is not immediately apparent and may take up to 2 weeks to develop, and it may progress for 6 months after the incident [25–29]. The ulcer may have a raised red or yellow necrotic wound bed [1,12] and may be painful, and it tends to increase in size and depth, thereby deterring healing [1,12]. Compartment syndrome results in sequelae ranging from muscular changes to ischemic nerve damage that may result in functional loss of the extremity [27]. Reflex sympathetic dystrophy syndrome is caused by trauma to nerve complexes or soft tissue, resulting in a chronic and exaggerated inflammatory process that leaves the patient with limited function of the affected extremity [26].

Signs and symptoms of extravasation

Classic signs of extravasations include itching, pain, tightness, edema, blanching, and coolness at the site [25–27]. Not all patients experience discomfort [27]. Research demonstrates that pain, edema, and induration are unreliable indicators of extravasation [27]. Signs of extravasation may spare the insertion site but present instead anywhere along the entire length of the catheter and adjacent structures [27]. Over time, these symptoms may increase, and discoloration, induration, dry desquamation, or blistering of the skin may develop [25–27]. With extravasation caused by the use of a central vascular access device, signs may be evident at the subcutaneous tunnel or port pocket, neck, jaw, arm, and chest wall ipsilateral to the catheter [25,28,29].

Impaired wound healing in extravasation wounds

Extravasation wounds lack a significant inflammatory response and have little granulation formation and re-epithelialization, which characterizes normal wound healing [1,24]. On histologic examination, extravasation wounds show multiple changes in fibroblasts [1,12,24]. Myofibroblasts appear normal in the wound, but they may be dysfunctional, resulting in a lack of wound contraction [1,12].

Prevention of extravasation

The most important approach to extravasation is prevention. Prevention includes assessment and knowledge of the patient, vesicant potential of the drug, and administration of chemotherapy only by specially trained nurses [25–29]. The Oncology Nursing Society Chemotherapy and Biotherapy Guidelines (2001) describe detailed policies for chemotherapy administration and management of extravasation [25].

Treatment of extravasation

There is little agreement in the literature concerning treatment modalities, appropriate timing of interventions after injury, and recommendations for local wound care [24,25,27]. Many of the currently recommended therapies are based on anecdotal findings and limited experimental data [25,27]. Most authors agree that the sooner the treatment is initiated, the better the outcome will be [25,27]. Treatment for extravasation depends largely on the vesicant and whether an antidote exists to inactivate the infiltrated drug [24,25]. The study of antidotes in humans for the treatment of extravasation has been limited because of ethical reasons [24,25]. For most vesicants, no antidote exists [24,27]. Two drugs, hyaluronidase (Wydase) and phentolamine, which were previously used for treatment of extravasations, have been removed from the market, and no drugs have been identified as replacements [27,30]. Sodium bicarbonate, once believed to be an effective antidote for doxorubicin extravasation, is no longer recommended because it has been shown to actually increase toxicity [11]. Currently, isotonic sodium thiosulfate is the only antidote listed for treating chemotherapy extravasation in the Oncology Nursing Society Chemotherapy and Biotherapy Guidelines [25]. Table 3 lists chemotherapy vesicants, antidotes, and nursing measures.

The efficacy of using cold or warm compresses and elevation after extravasation has not been established [11,24,27]. Despite the unproven benefits of these interventions, they increase patient comfort and should be used on an intermittent basis for as long as they can be tolerated [11,25]. Pressure on the extravasation site should be avoided because it can spread the vesicant over a larger surface area [11,25,27].

Treatment for ulceration may include early or late surgical debridement with subsequent use of a biologic dressing and or skin graft [11,24]. Biologic dressings are skin substitutes grown in the laboratory from human neonate and foreskin cells and collagen (eg, Apligraf, Dermagraft) [31,32]. Surgical excision is generally indicated if pain persists after 3 to 7 days [11,24]. Most surgeons opt for a conservative approach in the absence of these symptoms [24]. However, if swelling, erythema, and pain without ulceration persist after conservative therapy, then debridement should be strongly considered [11,24,26].

Table 3
Chemotherapy vesicants, antidotes, and nursing measures

	Antidote	Nursing measures
Alkylating agents		
Mechlorethamine hydrochloride (nitrogen mustard)	Isotonic sodium thiosulfate	1. Sodium thiosulfate neutralizes nitrogen mustard 2. Heat and cold have not been proven 3. Time is essential in treating extravasation
Cisplatin (Platinol)	Isotonic sodium thiosulfate	Vesicant potential seen when a concentration of more than 20 cc 0.5 mg/ml extravasates. If less than this, drug is an irritant; no treatment is recommended.
Antitumor antibiotics		
Doxorubicin (Adriamycin)	None	1. Extravasations of less than 1–2 cc often heal spontaneously. If greater than 3 cc, ulceration often results. 2. Apply cold pad with circulating ice water, ice pack, or cryogel pack for 15–20 min at least four times per day for the first 24–48 h. 3. Protect area from sunlight. 4. Some studies suggest dimethyl sulfoxide (DMSO) applied topically to site every 6 h is beneficial; other studies show delayed healing with DMSO.
Daunorubicin (Cerubidine)	None	1. Little information known 2. In mouse experiments, topical DMSO affords some benefit
Mitomycin	None	1. Protect area of extravasation from sunlight 2. Delayed skin reactions have occurred in areas far from original IV site 3. Some studies show benefit with DMSO; more studies are needed
Dactinomycin (actinomycin-D, Cosmegen)	None	1. Apply ice to increase comfort at site 2. Heat may enhance tissue damage 3. Elevate site for 48 h, then resume normal activity
Mitoxantrone (Novantrone)	Unknown	1. Antidote or local-care measures are unknown 2. Ulceration rare unless concentrated dose infiltrates

Epirubicin, Ellence Idarubicin (Idamycin) Esorubicin	None	1. Antidote and local-care measures are unknown 2. Cold, DMSO, and corticosteroids are ineffective based on experiments with mice 3. Esorubicin phlebitis is common
Vinca alkaloids or microtubular inhibiting agents		
Vincristine (Oncovin)	None	1. Apply heat for 15–20 min at least four times per day for the first 24–48 h 2. This method of treatment is very effective for rapid absorption of drug
Vinblastine (Velban)	None	Same as above
Vindesine (not available in United States)	None	Same as above
Vinorelbine (Navelbine)	None	1. Same as cited for vincristine and vinblastine 2. Vinorelbine is a moderate vesicant 3. Manufacturer recommends administering drug over 6–10 min into side port of free-flowing IV closest to the IV bag followed by a flush of 75–125 mL. IV solution to reduce incidence of phlebitis and severe back pain
Taxanes		
Paclitaxel (Taxol)	None	1. Recent documentation of vesicant potential 2. Paclitaxel has rare vesicant potential (probably caused by dilution in 500-cc diluent) 3. Ice has been effective in decreasing local tissue damage in a mouse model 4. Apply ice pack for 15–20 min at least four times per day for the first 24 hours

From Brown KA, Esper P, Kelleher LO, et al, editors. Chemotherapy and biotherapy guidelines and recommendations for practice. Philadelphia: Oncology Nursing Society; 2001. p. 60–1; with permission.

Local wound care should include cleansing with normal saline (as described earlier) and the use of hydrogel dressings [1,11]. Hydrogel dressings are believed to aid autolytic debridement of necrotic tissue, prevent dehydration of damaged tissue, and further limit devitalization of the exposed dermis [1,11]. Because the full extent of tissue damage may not initially be evident, the surrounding skin should be treated as potentially friable, and tape should be avoided. Dressings should be secured with nonadhesive stabilizing devices such as tubular stretch gauze, described previously. The use of silver sulfadiazine is recommended when open or closed bullae are present and when there is a risk of infection caused by neutropenia [11]. Silver sulfadiazine provides wide-spectrum antimicrobial activity and must be applied twice per day because the silver ions are inactivated after 12 hours [11]. Prolonged use of silver sulfadiazine may result in the development of resistant organisms [22,32]. Data support limiting the treatment with topical antibiotics to no longer than 2 weeks [19]. The newer antimicrobial dressings containing silver may have a similar indication as silver sulfadiazine for these wounds. Examples of silver-impregnated antimicrobial dressings include Acticoat (Smith & Nephew), Arglaes (Medline Industries, Inc), and Aguacel AG (Convatec) [32].

New directions in treatment of extravasation wounds

In animal models, the use of hyperbaric oxygen therapy in wounds with doxorubicin extravasation demonstrated beneficial effects on healing but potentiated the toxicity of doxorubicin [24]. Clinicians have also reported that the off-label use of a subcutaneous granulocyte macrophage colony-stimulating agent (eg, Sargamostin) has demonstrated effective healing in doxorubicin and vincristine extravasations [24,33,34]. In previous animal models, granulocyte macrophage colony-stimulating has also demonstrated a beneficial effect on doxorubicin-induced tissue necrosis [24]. Granulocyte macrophage colony-stimulating enhances the migration and proliferation of endothelial cells and promotes keratinocyte growth [33,34].

Before starting vesicant chemotherapy, nurses should inform patients that extravasation is a known risk and that unusual sensations such as pain are not normal and should be reported immediately [28]. Patient education regarding the risk of extravasation should be reviewed and documented with each infusion [25,28]. If an extravasation should occur, nurses should follow their institutional policy and notify the physician of the incident [25,28]. Assessments should be ongoing and include close monitoring of the extravasation site, blood counts, and photographs [25,28].

Radiation: a brief overview

Radiation therapy (RT) is the use of high-energy x-rays or particles to treat disease [35]. RT is one of the oldest cancer treatments and more than 50% of cancer patients presently receive some form of radiation treatment, either preoperatively, postoperatively, or as a sole treatment [35,36]. Radiation is used to treat local or regional disease and, rarely, systemic disease [37].

Effects of radiation

Although improved radiation techniques and equipment have lessened both the incidence and severity of radiation skin reactions, patients are still experiencing radiation-induced injury [36,37]. Radiation injury is defined as morphologic and functional changes that can occur in noncancerous tissue as a direct result of ionizing radiation [36–38]. Ionizing radiation causes damage by means of free radicals and reactive oxygen intermediates that damage cellular components, including DNA [37,38]. Injury can range from mild skin reactions that are self-limiting to long-term chronic skin changes with necrosis and ulceration [36–38]. The incidence of chronic skin changes caused by radiation varies from 0% to 40%, depending on treatment variables [36,37].

Radiation beams penetrate the skin to reach the target area [35]. These effects are most evident in the epidermis, hair follicles, and sebaceous glands [11,36]. Box 1 lists factors that influence the degree of skin reaction with radiation. Previous literature [37,38] suggests that variations in tissue reactions to radiation may be related to individual characteristics because patients treated with identical radiotherapy schedules show a substantial variation in degrees of tissue reactions. Porock (1998) [38] explored potential predictors of radiation-induced skin reactions among women with breast cancer who had undergone lumpectomy followed by a standard radiation protocol. Chi square analysis revealed that many factors are associated with a more severe reaction, including personal histories, such as smoking, alcohol, and nutritional intake [38].

Histologically, morphologic cell changes result from the dose of radiation delivered [36,37]. Low doses of radiation produce changes mainly in the cell nucleus, whereas damage from high doses of radiation may cause a loss of the nuclear membrane resulting from direct cellular necrosis [36,37]. Patients treated with a high dose of radiation to the skin and large fractions are at greater risk of developing late skin effects [35–37].

Immediate and acute skin reactions

Because radiation beams must penetrate the skin to reach the target area, most patients will experience some degree of acute skin effects [35,36]. Side effects of RT may be divided into immediate (days to weeks), acute (2 to 3 weeks), and delayed (months to years) [36]. In the first 2 weeks, exposure to ionizing radiation exceeding 10 Gy (Gy, or gray, is the measure of radiation), produces local skin reactions characterized by mild erythema,

---

Box 1. Factors that influence the degree of skin reaction with radiation

- Site of treatment field (eg, reaction is worse in skin fold areas with friction such as the axilla, inframammary area, groin, and perineum)
- Total radiation dose
- Dose of daily fraction and radiation boost
- Type and level of energy of radiation used
- Use of chemotherapy and radiosensitizing agents:
  Dactinomycin, doxorubicin, methotrexate, 5-fluorouracil, and
      hydroxyurea may sensitize the basal cells to radiation.
      Patients who receive chemotherapy several months after RT
      may experience "radiation recall," in which a tissue reaction
      is produced within the previous treatment field.
      Dactinomycin and doxorubicin are known to cause radiation
      recall
- Nutritional status
- Individual differences among patients (eg, age and gender)

Data from Bruner DW, Bucholtz JD, Iwanota R, Strohl R, editors. Manual for radiation oncology nursing practice and education. Philadelphia: Oncology Nursing Society; 1998. p. 18.

---

edema, and pruritus [36]. With exposure to higher doses, more severe reactions will occur, including intense erythema, erosion, and superficial ulceration [36]. This acute reaction begins 2 to 7 days after treatment, peaks within 2 weeks, and gradually resolves [36]. Skin reactions result from necrosis of the rapidly proliferating cell lines in the epidermis, hair follicles, and sebaceous glands [36,37]. Immediate reactions are caused by inflammation, whereas acute reactions are caused by dilation of the vessels in the irradiated area [36].

If the total radiation dose does not exceed approximately 30 Gy, a dry desquamation phase occurs during the fourth or fifth week [36]. Dry desquamation is characterized by pruritus, scaling, and an increase in melanin pigment [36]. If the total radiation dose is 40 Gy or greater, moist desquamation will follow the erythema phase in the fourth week. Moist desquamation is characterized by bullous formation and potential shedding of the entire epidermis, with edema and fibrous exudate [36]. In the absence of infection, re-epithelialization begins in 10 days [36]. Ulcers may form at any time in the first 2 weeks after initiation of radiation; these ulcers usually heal but tend to recur as a direct result of necrosis of the epidermis [36,39].

Late skin effects

Late reactions are classified as those that occur six or more months after RT and are characterized by skin that is pigmented, dry from loss of sebaceous glands, and hairless [11,36]. Much of the collagen and sub-cutaneous adipose tissue is replaced by atypical fibroblasts and dense fibrous tissue that may cause induration of skin and limit movement. The skin is easily damaged, and this can lead to nonhealing wounds [1,36,39]. The incidence of wounds is estimated to be 3% to 10% across tissue sites [1]. A 10-year retrospective study by Landthaler [40] reported that radiation-induced ulcers appeared after a mean latency period of 8 years, 7 months. The frequency of ulcers increased with total dose of radiation and decreased with the increasing age of the patient. Characteristics of radiation wounds are listed in Box 2.

Assessment of patients who receive radiation should include evaluation of the pretreatment skin status and identification of potential risk factors listed in Box 1 [37,41]. The appearance of the skin should be assessed and documented before treatment and on each subsequent visit [37,41]. The Oncology Nursing Society has published a radiation therapy Patient Care Record [41], which includes assessment parameters and common toxicity criteria for patients receiving radiation therapy, including skin sensation and radiation dermatitis [37,41]. Table 4 lists the necessary components of education for patients who receive radiation treatment [37].

Box 2. Characteristics of radiation wounds

- Wounds vary in depth
- The wound bed is covered with fibropurulent material
- Wounds have raised red edges and a necrotic nonvascularized base
- Do not heal spontaneously because of a lack of functional fibroblasts and altered migratory ability of cells
- Wounds are unable to contract spontaneously
- Tissue remains relatively ischemic (patients are at an increased risk of infection and experience further delays in healing)
- May be painful

Data from McDonald AE. Skin ulceration. In: Groenwald S, Frogge MH, Goodman M, and Yarbro CH, editors. Cancer symptom management. Boston: Jones and Bartlett Publishers; 1996. p. 368–9; and Black JM, Black SB. Complex wounds. In: Barnoski S, Ayello EA, editors. Wound care essentials practice principles. Philadelphia: Lippincott Williams & Wilkins; 2003. p. 378.

Table 4
Care of radiation skin and wounds

Issue	Intervention	Patient and family education
Cleansing	Gentle cleansing with water, normal saline, or a mild soap rinsed thoroughly to avoid excessive irritation.	Wash skin gently with a mild soap and lukewarm water
Moisturizing	Hydrophilic preparations absorb water and act as mild lubricants (eg, Eucerin, Beiersdorf; Lubriderm; Pfizer)	Regular skin moisturizing Identify which sites are high risks for skin reactions Avoid irritants (eg, deodorants, soaps, lotions, perfumes other than recommended by the physician or nurse)
Protection	Protective ointments or gels are effective for protecting dry lesions (Aquaphor, Beiersdorf; A+D Ointment, Schering-Plough)	Avoid friction (e.g. skin surfaces rubbing together, clothing rubbing against skin) Avoid products containing alcohol or menthol because they remove natural lipids from the skin and may worsen the reaction Use an electric razor only Avoid sun exposure Regular use of a sunscreen with an SPF of 15 or higher if expected to be in direct sun exposure for more than 15 minutes
Dry Desquamation	Hydrophilic preparations protect and lubricate scaly or flaking skin resulting from loss of sweat and sebaceous glands Hydrogel dressings serve to rehydrate the skin (Carrasyn Gel, Carrington Laboratories; aloe vera gel; Biafine, Medix Pharmaceuticals)	Report signs and symptoms of dry and moist desquamation
Pruritus	The following products can be used to decease pruritus: Colloidal oatmeal bath (Aveeno Bath, Rydelle Laboratories) Mild steroids such as hydrocortisone cream 1% can be applied to irritated, inflamed skin	Use of antipruritic medications Discontinue use of hydrocortisone cream after symptoms resolve

	Do not use on moist skin reactions because it may enhance infection	
Moist Desquamation	Cornstarch can be applied to intact skin, especially skin folds, to decrease excess moisture and itching; however, cornstarch is discouraged when areas of moist desquamation are present because it enhances bacterial and fungal growth	
	Can be treated with topical soaks (eg, Domeboro, Bayer Corporation) for 15–20 min, three to four times per day. follow with a gel or lotion such as Aquaphor or Eucerin	Treatment break may be indicated if moist desquamation is severe
Dressings	Wet and painful wounds should be covered to decrease pain, control fluid loss, prevent evaporation, and reduce the risk of infection	Use of dressings
	Dressings maintain a moist environment that enhances reepithelialization and facilitates autolytic debridement Examples: hydrogels, hydrocolloids, and absorptive dressings; frequency of dressing change varies between products; do not use dry gauze dressings because they can adhere to the wound.	Hydrocolloids should be removed with gentle technique to prevent the stripping of healing skin
Antibiotics	Topical antibiotics are indicated if proven by wound culture Topical silver sulfadiazine 1% is recommended by some clinicians to cover gram-positive and gram-negative organisms and Candida albicans; systemic antibiotic therapy is warranted if the area does not heal.	Report signs and symptoms of infection Increased wound pain may indicate infection
Xerosis	Localized xerosis may over the long term develop; mild soaps and bath oils may be used during bathing Neutral soaps have a pH of less than 7.5 (eg, Basis, Beiersdorf; Lowila Cake, Westwood-Squibb) Skin cleansers formulated to cleanse and moisturize while preserving normal skin pH (eg, Aloe Vesta 2-n-1 Body Wash and Shampoo, Convatec)	Regularly lubricate the skin to prevent fissures, and keep the skin pliable Dry skin lotions, creams

(continued on next page)

Table 4 (*continued*)

Issue	Intervention	Patient and family education
Severe radiation wounds	Lubricants such as petrolatum and mineral oil are generally more effective but less pleasing to patients Recalcitrant irradiation wounds may require skin grafting, (eg; flap) involving excision of the wound and reconstruction with arterialized tissues to bring in a new blood supply. Certain dressings used for thermal burns may be applied to the radiation wounds and donor graft sites: Biosynthetic and synthetic: (eg, Biobrane, Opsite, and Tegaderm); artificial skin: (eg, Integra); bioengineered skin: (Apligraf)	Maintain good nutritional intake to aid wound healing

Data from Mendelsohn FA, Divino CM, Reis ED, et al. Wound care after radiation therapy. Adv Wound Care 2002;15:216–24; and Bruner DW, Bucholtz, JD, Iwanota R, et al, editors. Manual for radiation oncology nursing practice and education. Philadelphia: Oncology Nursing Society; 1998. p. 1–80.

Treatment of radiation-induced skin injury

Treatment of specific skin reactions varies greatly from institution to institution [11,35–37]. To date, little research is available showing that one skin care agent can prevent radiation skin reaction or increase healing time better than another [11,35,37]. Nursing care is aimed at minimizing discomfort, promoting healing, and minimizing complications of radiation therapy [35,36]. Wounds caused by radiation therapy are typically difficult and slow to heal [36,39]. Treatment of wounds following radiation should begin by first, ruling out a recurrent or new malignancy in the area [36,39]. The principles of burn therapy have been applied to the management of severe radiation reactions, which may by painful, draining, and involve extensive desquamation [11,36,41]. Certain dressings that are used for thermal burns, such as biologic dressings, may be applied to the radiation wounds and donor grafts [11,36,39]. Recalcitrant radiation wounds may require skin grafting methods such as a flap, involving excision of the wound and reconstruction with arterialized tissues to bring in a new blood supply [12]. However, adherence to principles of moist wound therapy, proper wound cleansing, as described earlier, and prevention of infection may promote closure of these wounds without surgical intervention [11,36]. Table 5 provides a summary of care following radiation-induced skin injury.

Current research with radiation skin injury

Alternative treatment strategies being investigated for radiation-induced skin injury include the use of growth factors, cytokines, antioxidants, topical steroids, non-steroidal anti-inflammatory preparations, aloe vera, and lasers [37,42]. Table 5 summarizes experimental treatment strategies for radiation-induced skin injury.

Summary

As cancer continues to represent a major health problem in the United States and in other developed countries, MCWs will continue to represent a complex problem for patients and health care professionals alike. Goals of care may range from healing to palliation, depending on the underlying pathology and patient preferences regarding their personal goals of wound or disease management. Palliative wound care should focus on patient comfort and quality of life as the goals, instead of wound. As evidence related to wound healing, products, and technology continues to increase, nurses can be at the forefront of putting into practice the science of wound healing for the benefit of patients.

Table 5
Experimental treatment strategies for radiation-induced skin injury

Agent	Category	Mechanism of action	Protocol	Results
TGF-β1	Growth factor	A protein that has an important role in wound healing; increases angiogenesis, probably by modulating macrophages to release factors that lead to revascularization.	Using a rat model, evaluated the effect of TGF-1 on wound healing and random flap survival in chronic irradiation.	TGF-β1 improves wound healing and random flap survival in radiated and nonirradiated rat skin.
			Studied the effect of TGF-1 on healing of radiation-impaired wounds using a guinea pig model.	Statistically significant increases in wound bursting strength were seen in irradiated wounds; total dose of TGF-1 must be monitored to avoid effects opposite to those desired.
TGF-β1 inhibitors	Cytokine	Demonstrated to decrease the amount of late radiation fibrosis.	Studies in vitro research of human fibroblasts and keratinocytes or mice models. New data obtained from animal studies and human fibroblast research.	May be effective in reducing longstanding radiation fibrosis.
Orgotein	Antioxidant	A metalloprotein that may have protective effect on radiation cystitis and proctitis.	Randomize trial with 19 patients	Showed no effect; trial stopped early due to local reaction of subcutaneous infiltration
			Evaluated the use of orgotein in patients with bladder cancer.	Orgotein effective in decreasing acute radiation-induced damage and in preventing the appearance of more delayed disorders.

			Study	Results
			Investigated the radioprotective effects of orgotein on normal skin and malignant murine tissue in vivo.	No effects of orgotein were seen on tumor radiation response; however, a protective effect was observed on normal skin for early and permanent damage. More rapid tissue healing was noted in the instance of early damage.
Topical vitamin C solution	Antioxidant	An antioxidant that has the potential to protect nonmalignant tissue from radiation and improve collagen synthesis.	Administered ascorbic acid to 50 mice before whole-body radiation.	Significantly increased the dose of radiation required to obtain skin desquamation.
			Evaluated the value of topical ascorbic acid in preventing radiation dermatitis in patients with primary or metastatic brain tumors requiring external beam radiation.	Unable to demonstrate a significant effect which is not surprising, since little ascorbic acid is absorbed topically.
Topical corticosteroids	Anti-inflammatory	Have been shown to have an anti-inflammatory effect in radiation dermatitis.	Two different steroid creams were compared in patients receiving radiation for breast cancer.	Both groups of patients derived benefit from soothing effects, but a dramatic difference in intensity of reactions was noted; hydrocortisone is superior to clobetasone butyrate, but neither cream was efficacious enough to be recommended as a first choice for initial treatment.

(continued on next page)

Table 5 (*continued*)

Agent	Category	Mechanism of action	Protocol	Results
			Examined effects of 1% topical indomethacin and 1% topical hydrocortisone applied before and during radiation.	Patients treated with indomethacin developed more severe erythematous reactions after 5 weeks of starting therapy. Hydrocortisone applied at the time of radiation produces lasting beneficial effects and can still be seen several weeks after application is discontinued.
Aloe vera gel	Prophylactic	Several compounds have been discovered in the aloe vera plant may help to decrease inflammation. Known to possess antibacterial and antifungal properties.	Conducted two Phase III randomized trials that compared aloe vera gel with placebo or no treatment.	Neither trial showed any significant benefit from use of aloe vera. The distributions of maximum dermatitis severity scores were nearly identical in both treatment arms, regardless of whether scored by patient or health care provider.
			Prospective, randomized trial to determine whether the use of mild soap and aloe vera gel versus mild soap alone would decrease the incidence of skin reactions in patients undergoing radiation therapy.	At low cumulative does levels 2,700 Gy, no difference existed in the effect of adding aloe vera. When the cumulative dose >2,700 Gy, the median time was five weeks prior to any skin changes in the aloe/soap arm versus three weeks in the soap only arm. When the cumulative dose increases over time, there seems to be a protective effect of adding aloe to the soap regimen.

Helium-neon laser irradiation	Laser	Laser treatments can enhance metabolic pathways by several different mechanisms. Evidence exists for the possible improvement of skin circulation and induction of angiogenesis.	Patients with recalcitrant radiation ulcers of the skin after mastectomy were treated with a helium laser 3 times weekly.	Low intensity helium-neon laser irradiation was demonstrated to have a beneficial effect on impaired wound healing of recalcitrant skin ulcers after radiation therapy.
GM-CSF	Colony stimulating factor	Believed to stimulate wound healing by various processes; most importantly, its stimulation of proliferation and differentiation of basal epithelial stem cells.	Investigated the effectiveness of GM-CSF impregnated gauze along with steroid cream versus steroid cram alone in 61 patients receiving radiation for vulvar carcinoma in preventing or healing radiation-induced dermatitis.	The use of GM-CSF showed statistically significant reduction in the duration of symptoms, the healing period of dermatitis, and the pain and severity of dermatitis. No cutaneous or systemic toxicities or allergic reactions were noted.

Abbreviations: GM-CSF, granulocyte macrophage colony-stimulating factor; TGF, transforming growth factor.

Data from Mendelsohn FA, Divino CM, Reis ED, et al. Wound care after radiation therapy. Adv Wound Care 2002;15(5):216–24; and Olsen DL, Raub W, Bradley C, et al. The effect of aloe vera gel/mild soap alone in preventing skin reactions in patients undergoing radiation therapy. Clin J Oncol Nurs 2001;28:1–9.

References

[1] McDonald AE. Skin ulceration. In: Groenwald SL, Frogge MH, Goodman M, et al, editors. Cancer symptom management. Boston: Jones and Bartlettt Publishers; 1996. p. 364–81.

[2] Haisfield-Wolfe ME, Baxendale-Cox LM. Staging of malignant cutaneous wounds: a pilot study. Oncol Nurs Forum 1999;26(6):1–12.

[3] Trent JT, Kirsner RS. Wounds and malignancy. Adv Skin Wound Care 2003;16(1):31–4.

[4] Haisfield-Wolfe ME, Rund C. A nursing protocol for the management of perineal-rectal skin alterations. Clin J Oncol Nurs 2000;4(1):1–12.

[5] Haisfield-Wolfe ME. Malignant cutaneous wounds: a management protocol. Ostomy Wound Manage 1997;43(1):56–66.

[6] Baharestani MM. Quality of life and ethical issues. In: Barnoski S, Ayello EA, editors. Wound care essentials practice principles. Philadelphia: Lippincott, Williams, and Wilkins; 2003. p. 2–18.

[7] Bauer C, Gerlach MA. Care of metastatic skin lesions. J Wound Ostomy Continence Nurs 2000;27(4):247–51.

[8] Jones V, Bale S, Harding K. Acute and chronic wound healing. In: Barnoski S, Ayello EA, editors. Wound care essentials practice principles. Philadelphia: Lippincott, Williams, and Wilkins; 2003. p. 61–78.

[9] Smeltzer SC, Bare BG. Postoperative nursing management. In: Textbook of medical-surgical nursing. 9th edition. Philadelphia: Lippincott, Williams, and Wilkins; 2000. p. 347–70.

[10] Bacilious N, Disa JJ. Managing the oncology wound: reconstructive issues in breast cancer. Ostomy Wound Manage 2000;46(Suppl 1A):S32–6 Jan.

[11] Goldberg MT, McGinn-Byer P. Oncology-related skin damage. In: Bryant RA, editor. Acute and chronic wounds. 2nd edition. St Louis (MO): Mosby; 2000. p. 367–86.

[12] Araujo T, Kirsner RS. Atypical wounds in acute and chronic wounds. In: Barnoski S, Ayello EA, editors. Wound care essentials practice principles. Philadelphia: Lippincott, Williams, and Wilkins; 2003. p. 381–98.

[13] Albert MR, Weinstock MA. Keratinocyte carcinoma. CA Cancer J Clin 2003;53(5):292–302.

[14] Goodman M, Hilderley L, Purls S. Integumentary and mucous membrane alteration. In: Groenwald S, Hansen-Frogge M, Goodman M, et al, editors. Cancer nursing: principles and practice. 4th edition. Boston: Jones and Bartlet; 1997. p. 768–822.

[15] Moore S. Cutaneous metastatic breast cancer. Clin J Oncol Nurs 2002;6(5):255–60.

[16] Schiech L. Malignant cutaneous wounds. Clin J Oncol Nurs 2002;6(5):305–9.

[17] Woodward L, Haisfield-Wolfe ME. Management of a patient with a malignant cutaneous tumor. Journal Wound Ostomy Continence Nurs 2003;30(4):231–6.

[18] Bauer C. Metastatic skin lesions. In: Milne CT, Corbett LQ, Dubuc DL, editors. Wound, ostomy, and continence nursing secrets. Philadelphia: Hanley & Belfus, Inc.; 2003. p. 231–3.

[19] Gardner SE, Frantz RA. Wound bioburden. In: Barnoski S, Ayello EA, editors. Wound care essentials practice principles. Philadelphia: Lippincott, Williams, and Wilkins; 2003. p. 91–116.

[20] Lawrence JC, Lilly HA, Kisdon A. Malodour and dressings containing active charcoal. Proceedings of the 2nd Europena Conference on Advances in Wound Management. October 20–23, 1992. Harrogate, UK. p. 73–4.

[21] Poteete V. Case study: eliminating odors from wounds. Decubitus 1993;6(4):43–5.

[22] McGuckin M, Goldman R, Bolton L, et al. The clinical relevance of microbiology in acute and chronic wounds. Adv Skin Wound Care 2003;16(1):12–23.

[23] Wilson R. Massive tissue loss: burns. In: Bryant RA, editor. Acute and chronic wounds. 2nd edition. St Louis (MO): Mosby; 2000. p. 197–209.

[24] Schrijvers DL. Extravasation: a dreaded complication of chemotherapy. Ann Oncol 2003; 14(Suppl 3):Siii26–30.

[25] Brown KA, Esper P, Kelleher LO, et al, editors. Chemotherapy and biotherapy guidelines and recommendations for practice. Philadelphia: Oncology Nursing Society; 2001. p. 1–220.

[26] Roth D. Extravasation injuries of peripheral veins a basis for litigation. Journal of Vascular Access Devices 2003;Spring:13–9.

[27] Hadaway LC. I.V. infiltration: not just a peripheral problem. Nursing 2002;August:1–9.

[28] Schulmeister L. Chemotherapy extravasation from implanted ports. Clin J Oncol Nurs 2000; 27(3):1–14.

[29] Masoorli S. Extravasation injuries associated with the use of central vascular access devices. Journal of Vascular Access Devices 2003;Spring:21–3.

[30] Oncology Nursing Society. What can I use for an extravasation now that Wydase is no longer available? Available at: http://www.ons.org/xp6/ONS/Information.xml/About_ ONS.xml/FAQ.xml. Accessed February 19, 2004.

[31] Novartis. PDF Apligraf. Available at: http://www.pharma.us.novartis.com/product/pi/pdf/ apligraf.pdf. Accessed February 21, 2004.

[32] Barnoski S, Ayello E. Wound treatment options in acute and chronic wounds. In: Barnoski S, Ayello EA, editors. Wound care essentials practice principles. Philadelphia: Lippincott, Williams, and Wilkins; 2003. p. 127–56.

[33] Bushel PC, Forgey AN, Browning-Grape F, et al. Granulocyte macrophage colony-stimulating factor: current practice and novel approaches. Clin J Oncol Nurs 2002;6(4):1–13.

[34] Lawrence S. GM-CSF for extravasation of doxorubicin and vincristine [abstract 114]. Available at: http://www.ons.org/xp6/ONS/Abstracts.xml/Abstracts_2002.xml/ Full_Abstract_Contents/2002_114.xml. Accessed February 26, 2004.

[35] Strohl RA. Radiation skin reactions. Progressions 1998;1(3):3–9.

[36] Mendelsohn FA, Divino CM, Reis ED, et al. Wound care after radiation therapy: advances in skin and wound care. Adv Wound Care 2002;15(5):216–24.

[37] Bruner DW, Bucholtz JD, Iwanota R, et al, editors. Manual for radiation oncology nursing practice and education. Philadelphia: Oncology Nursing Society; 1998. p. 1–80.

[38] Porock D. Predicting severity of radiation skin reactions in women with breast cancer. Available at: http://www.ons.org/xp6/ONS/Convention.xml/Abstracts.xml/Abstracts_1998.xml/ Full_Abstract_Contents/Number_19984.xml. Accessed February 21, 2004.

[39] Black JM, Black SB. Complex wounds: in acute and chronic wounds. In: Barnoski S, Ayello EA, editors. Wound care essentials practice principles. Philadelphia: Lippincott, Williams, and, Wilkins; 2003. p. 367–80.

[40] Landthaler M, Hagspiel HJ, Braun F. Late irradiation damage to skin x-ray radiation therapy of cutaneous tumors. Arch Dermatol 1995;131(2):182–6.

[41] Catlin-Hugh C, Haas M, Pollock V, editors. Radiation therapy patient care record: a tool for documenting nursing care. Philadelphia: Oncology Nursing Society; 2002. p. 1–21.

[42] Olsen DL, Raub W, Bradley C, et al. The effect of aloe vera gel/mild soap versus mild soap alone in preventing skin reactions in patients undergoing radiation therapy. Clin J Oncol Nurs 2001;28(3):1–9.

NURSING
CLINICS
OF NORTH AMERICA

Nurs Clin N Am 40 (2005) 325–335

The Challenges of Obesity and Skin Integrity

Susan Gallagher, RN, CWOCN, MA, MSN, PhD

Houston, TX, USA

The challenge of caring for the overweight patient lies in the special care and knowledge that are required for a meaningful clinical outcome. Obesity is associated with numerous coexisting conditions such as diabetes, situational depression, hypertension, soft tissue infection, some cancers, and impaired circulation, which could interfere with the patient's level of health, in general, and skin care, specifically. Some authors believe that from the onset of these conditions, the obese patient is at a disadvantage because diagnosis is difficult, and procedures are technically more complicated [1]. Many hospitals report concerns about inadequate equipment, policies, and personnel to accommodate the needs of larger patients, and skin care becomes a clinical challenge in many cases. The skin, which is the largest organ of the body, is at particular risk for injury during hospitalization, especially in the presence of obesity. Demographics, the meaning of obesity, and factors that place the patient at particular risk for skin injury are described in this article. Prevention of common and predictable skin breakdown is discussed. Early assessment and intervention of skin injury, along with the value of an interdisciplinary approach, and legal implications are reviewed.

Changing demographics

Sixty-seven percent of Americans are overweight, and 10% to 15% are considered obese [2]. Six percent to 10% are morbidly obese, with a body mass index greater than 40 [3]. Americans spend nearly $33 billion annually in attempts to control or lose weight, whereas $100 billion is spent on obesity-related health problems. Despite widespread concern on all levels, Americans continue to gain weight. Obesity is a factor in five of the ten

E-mail address: susanmgsm@aol.com

leading causes of death [4] and is considered the second most common cause of preventable deaths in the United States [5].

The meaning of obesity

Obesity is the term assigned by the National Institutes of Health to describe the physical condition discussed in this article. Obesity, according to the National Institutes of Health, is simply a diagnostic category that represents a complex and multifactorial disease [6]; yet, in popular culture, even this diagnostic, clinical term holds a negative tone.

Obese Americans chose neither to be overweight nor to experience widespread prejudice and discrimination [7]. Prejudice is described as a prejudgment, whereas discrimination refers to an action based on this prejudgment. Overweight Americans experience both. Attitudes toward obesity are formed at a very young age; for example, children as young as 6 describe silhouettes of obese children as lazy, stupid, and ugly. This research suggests that prejudice toward the obese child is observed regardless of race or socioeconomic status [8]. Additionally, health care clinicians are also often biased against the larger patient [9], as are obese persons themselves [10]. Health care clinicians and organizations need to ensure a safe haven from obesity-related prejudice and discrimination [11].

There is widespread misunderstanding about the causes of obesity. What is understood is that weight gain occurs when intake, meaning food, exceeds output, meaning activity. However, the real mystery behind balancing body weight depends on many other factors. Genetics, gender, physiology, biochemistry, neuroscience, as well as cultural, environmental and psychosocial factors influence weight and its regulation [12]. Patients are best served when clinicians recognize obesity as the chronic condition that it is, making every effort to eliminate a culture of prejudice and discrimination.

The concern over prejudice and discrimination is that these emotions pose barriers to care regardless of practice setting or professional discipline. The overwhelming misunderstanding of obesity is likely to interfere with preplanning efforts, access to services, and resource allocation. Although this misunderstanding is not universal, it is pervasive enough to pose obstacles, and clinicians interested in making changes will need to recognize and overcome these barriers.

Skin and wound considerations

Skin and wound complications are immobility-related conditions that extend the need for clinical intervention regardless of the practice setting [13]. Clinicians provide the best service and assessment when they are familiar with common obesity-related complications, thus modifying care plans and clinical intervention to address or prevent complications.

Pressure ulcer precautions

Pressure ulcers develop because of a number of predisposing factors, but unrelieved pressure, friction, and shear present the three contributing causes (see the article by Maklebust elsewhere in this issue). Pressure ulcers typically occur over a bony prominence. Pressure ulcer staging is dependent on the depth of damage to the underlying tissue. In addition, obese patients can be at risk for atypical or unusual pressure ulcers, which can occur as a result of pressure within skin folds, tubes or catheters, or from an ill-fitting chair or wheelchair.

Pressure within skin folds can be sufficient to cause skin breakdown. Tubes and catheters burrow into skin folds, which can further erode the skin surface. Pressure from side rails and armrests not designed to accommodate a larger person can cause pressure ulcers on the patient's hips. Consider properly sized equipment that ensures sufficient space between the patient and the sides of the equipment. Additionally, the patient needs to be repositioned at least once every 2 hours, as do tubes and catheters. Tubes should be placed so that the patient does not rest on them. If this becomes difficult, tube and catheter holders may be helpful in this step. In the event that the patient has a large abdominal panniculus, it also must be repositioned to prevent pressure injury beneath the panniculus. Patients who are alert are able to physically lift the pannus off the suprapubic area. The weak, sedated or unconscious patient could be placed in the sidelying position in which the nurse can lift the pannus away from the underlying skin surface, allowing air to flow to the regions while relieving pressure. Use of rotation therapy is often regarded as the standard of care for certain pulmonary situations; however, it can also serve to ensure sufficient repositioning for a very large patient who otherwise may pose a realistic challenge to frequent turning. Despite the value of rotation therapy in prevention and treatment of skin injury among the obese patient, it is necessary to take precautions to prevent friction and shear. Correct pressure settings, fitting the patient to the appropriately sized surface, and assessment for skin changes can provide these precautions.

Candidiasis

Candida albicans thrives in a dark, moist environment, such as within skin folds. It is a normal inhabitant of the mouth, gastrointestinal tract, and vagina. *C. albicans* is one of the most common species found among human beings. Factors that contribute to candidiasis include immunocompromised states, diabetes mellitus, infection, chronic steroid use, hyperhidrosis, and obesity.

For assessment purposes, candidiasis is characterized by scaling erythema and, in some cases, small pustular lesions exist. Patients often complain of itching or burning and often scratch the skin surface, further compromising skin integrity, which can lead to a secondary bacterial invasion. Without intervention, this condition can lead to fissuring and maceration.

Candidiasis is manageable by using several approaches based on the severity of the situation. The first strategy is to eliminate excess moisture such as perspiration, incontinence, and wound drainage. If the patient complains of a moist skin surface, initially, an antifungal powder can be applied to clean, completely dry skin. For a dry, flaking surface, an antifungal cream can be helpful. To help soothe and cleanse affected skin, a soak or compress of Burrow's solution (aluminum acetate) can be applied for 15 to 20 minutes twice per day. Another remedy suggests using a 1% solution of acetic acid (10 mL of vinegar to 1 quart of water) as a soak or compress. If the condition does not improve within 24 hours, consider reassessing the condition because many skin conditions mimic one another [2].

Incontinence dermatitis

Moisture is a risk factor in skin breakdown; therefore, incontinence can complicate skin integrity. The patient may experience incontinence for the first time when hospitalized. This may be caused by medication, a delay in locating enough caregivers to assist the patient, or simply because the patient cannot reach a commode in time to prevent an incontinent episode. Physically compromised patients may be reluctant to ask for assistance with hygiene. Maintaining clean, dry skin is our objective, and if the patient needs assistance in this effort, caregivers must remind patients that our goal is to serve their needs and we can offer help in this respect.

After each incontinent episode, clean the entire affected area with an incontinence cleanser and then rinse and dry the area. Patients report that drying the buttocks, perineal area, and between folds with an institutionally approved blow dryer on the cool setting is more comfortable than towel drying. This technique may be less traumatic to the outermost layer of skin; however, again the patient may require assistance to reach this area.

If, despite preventive efforts, skin breakdown occurs, an aggressive plan of care is indicated. A moisture barrier ointment can serve as a protective barrier to chemicals in urine or stool. Few moisture barrier ointments adhere to weeping or moist areas of superficial breakdown. A light coat of protective powder applied to the moist areas may increase adherence of the moisture barrier ointment, thus more completely protecting the skin surface from the irritating chemicals found in stool and urine.

Surgical wounds

Surgical wounds are expected to create a watertight seal within 24 hours; however, wound healing can be delayed in some obese patients because of interference with the normal wound healing process. Blood supply to fatty tissue may be insufficient to provide an adequate amount of oxygen and nutrients. Wound healing may also be delayed if the patient has a diet that lacks essential vitamins and nutrients or if the wound is within a skin fold, where excess moisture and bacteria can accumulate. Furthermore, the excess body fat also increases the tension at the wound edges, making the wounds prone to dehiscence [14].

Increasing numbers of obese patients require abdominoplasty, especially after extensive weight loss associated with Roux-en-Y gastric bypass [15]. Abdominoplasty is a reconstructive surgical procedure intended to correct a problematic abdominal pannus and associated comorbidities. A large abdominal pannus, sometimes called an abdominal apron, is associated with cutaneous inflammation such as panniculitis, cellulitis, intertriginous dermatitis, skin abscesses, gangrene, excoriation, or folliculitis. Other concerns related to the pannus include back pain, lymphedema, ambulatory difficulty, and stress incontinence [16]. Abdominal panniculectomy and reconstructive abdominal surgery may be performed to alleviate these associated conditions. Wound care experts can be instrumental in providing documentation for reimbursement (Box 1).

Removal of the pannus will involve an incision extending from the xiphoid process to the pubic bone. There it meets a second, horizontal scar just above the pubic area to form what looks like an inverted letter "T." To create this T-shaped incision, the surgeon frees up fat and skin from the anterior abdomen. At that point, a large triangularly shaped area of loose skin and excess fat is carefully removed. The remaining tissue is then attached to the anterior abdominal wall and to itself. A number of procedures can be completed at the same time, such as exploratory

---

Box 1. Documentation for panniculectomy reimbursement

Third party payers have been known to refuse payment for abdominal panniculectomy for many reasons, one of which is the lack of photographic evidence coupled with a lack of clinical evidence. Therefore, it is prudent to document all observed and reported clinical symptoms that are associated with a large abdominal pannus, along with dated photographs [16]. Some payers require that the pannus hang down sufficiently so that it obscures the pubic area. Others reportedly look for intertrigo or other signs of inflammation under the pannus. Patient photographs, therefore, should include front, side, and under-surface views [16]. When all else fails, some patients have asked attorneys who specialize in reimbursement for bariatric needs to assist them in obtaining third party reimbursement [21].

laparotomy, revision of the primary surgery, and repair of abdominal wall and ventral hernia, each of which predisposes the patient to incisional challenges.

Early mobilization is critical in the recovery period. Many larger patients are able to turn, ambulate, and transfer soon after surgery, whereas others may have difficulty because of pain or sedation [17]. The physical therapist can assess the strength and endurance needs of the patient postoperatively. Wound dehiscence, seroma formation, and wound infection are common problems [18]. Drains are routinely placed after surgery, and it is important to observe for clotting of the drains or the unintentional removal of the drains by the patient. Infection can be a problem because many morbidly obese patients have associated medical problems, particularly type 2 diabetes mellitus, which contributes to delayed wound healing. Additionally, fatty tissue that is not excised can be devitalized, leading to fat necrosis and subsequent infection. Care should be taken when assessing the low mid point of the T in the abdominal incision because this is where a wound separation is most likely to occur [18]. All wounds should be kept clean and dry but especially those in skin folds. It will be important to contain any drainage, clean the area frequently with a nontoxic cleanser, and secure dry dressings to absorb excess moisture. In the event of a wound separation, patients can be taught to cleanse the opened area gently with a nontoxic wound cleanser, avoiding cytotoxic cleansers unless specifically indicated. Irregular body contours can present challenges in securing dressings. Flexible cloth tapes can be molded to the contours as necessary to ensure that the dressings are fixed securely to the intended area.

Freiberg [18] explains that some wound complications can be avoided or at least minimized by the use of an abdominal binder and later a girdle support. Abdominal binders should be worn for the first 4 weeks after surgery. Binders not only provide a degree of comfort to the patient but they minimize the shearing forces between the abdominal wall and abdominal skin. Binders are designed to control unnecessary edema and reduce ecchymosis. However, if the binder does not fit properly it can lead to skin breakdown, respiratory problems, or failure to comply with the plan of care. A clinical nurse specialist, as a member of the interdisciplinary team, can ensure that properly sized equipment is available. Assess the patient for skin and respiratory concerns when a binder is in place. Refer to the manufactures' guidelines to ensure safe use of the binder.

Legal considerations

From a legal perspective, larger Americans seldom bring attention to themselves. Many obese patients feel they are responsible for inadequate care because of their weight. However, in the past few years, size and weight acceptance advocates are asserting a legal right to equal, reasonable accommodation, demanding the same standards of care regardless of body size, weight, or configuration. The legal system provides a means for larger Americans to test this claim, and many times the claim is aimed at the health care community. Satisfied, informed consumers are less likely to file a claim against health care institutions or clinicians; therefore the failure to communicate is often at the heart of litigation, as is inadequate documentation. Legal mandates designed to protect patients are in place and are used nationwide for all types of negligence; therefore, it is in the best interests of any organization to recognize and understand the legal aspects of negligence when providing service to this high-risk patient population.

Negligence is a legal theory that applies to many medical malpractice cases. To win a negligence suit, the plaintiff must prove that four legal elements exist. The four legal elements of a claim are 1) duty, 2) breach of duty, 3) damages, and 4) causation. To ensure that the duty element is satisfied, a relationship must exist between the nurse (defendant) and the patient and a family member (plaintiff). The nurse holds a duty to perform consistently with an established standard of care.

A breach of duty exists when there has been a negligent departure from a recognized standard of care. A breach of duty, by definition, is the failure to do what the reasonable and prudent person possessing the same or similar skills and knowledge would do in the same or similar circumstances. If the court determines that a breach of duty has occurred, then it will be determined whether damages exist and to what extent. Despite the fact that the first three elements are present, it is still necessary for the plaintiff to prove that causation exists. The plaintiff must prove a direct causal relationship between the breach of duty and the alleged damages. This is done in two ways. The first is described by the notion of foreseeability, in which the plaintiff must prove that the defendant should have foreseen that the negligence could result in the alleged damages. The second way causation is proven is by making the following statement: in reasonable probability, the damages would not have occurred but for the negligence. In some parts of the country this is also stated by: the defendant's negligence was a substantial factor in causing the alleged damages.

Misunderstanding is sometimes at the heart of claims, for example, if the patient held an expectation that was not met by the health care institution or the nurses or an unexpected adverse outcome occurred. However, the occurrence of an adverse outcome does not prove negligence. Negligence must be proven using the four legal elements. Regardless, defending against a lawsuit can be economically and emotionally costly, and therefore avoiding lawsuits is a meaningful objective.

Communication can be interpreted in several ways. If the medical record suggests that there is lack of communication between nurses and other members of the health care team, this is considered a red flag and attorneys tend to investigate further. Clinicians on all levels must communicate, not only with each other but with the patient and family, when indicated. In the face of intervention that holds special risks, such as advanced skin and wound care, it is important to discuss this with the responsible party and document the discussion to that extent. Timely, accurate, and legible documentation of care and communication is imperative. In the event there are questions about what should be documented or how to document a special event, it may be in the nurse's best interest to speak to his or her risk manager. This is especially true in situations in which there are issues of inappropriate patient behavior.

Caring for larger patients is certainly more complex. Even without coexisting diagnoses or preadmission mobility issues, skin and wound care can be complicated sometimes simply because of the patient's body weight. Patients and caregivers are asked to perform tasks that they may be ill-equipped to accomplish. This raises questions of compliance. Sometimes the inability to carry out activities because of patient-related fear or apprehension is labeled noncompliance. It is important to try to differentiate this from a patient's refusal to participate in care; for example, a patient may refuse to ambulate for fear of falling, compared with a patient who refuses a physical therapy appointment because it coincides with a special television program. Understanding the difference is challenging in itself.

From a legal perspective, the issue of compliance is an important factor. Certainly, such issues pose documentation challenges. Again, in the case of failure to participate in care, the nurse may need to organize a team conference that would include the risk manager or hospital attorney. This is especially true if the health-defeating behavior affects the clinical outcome. Perhaps the team will discover that the seeming noncompliance is fear of the respective activity, in which case the support of a physical or occupational therapist, clinical social worker, or a psychologist would be necessary. However, if care concerns are not resolved in the team conference, the risk manager can direct the best method to document the situation. This step may protect the nurse and the institution from a lengthy legal encounter.

Clinical experts

The value of an interdisciplinary approach cannot be overlooked. Pharmacists, physical and respiratory therapists, physicians, and clinical nurse specialists are clinical experts who can be essential in planning care. Each member of the team brings a unique and important perspective. For example, consider the patient who undergoes removal of a 40-pound panniculus. This painful procedure could lead to immobility challenges and subsequent skin issues. The physical therapist may have ideas for mobilizing a patient who is otherwise immobile because of his body weight, pain, or sedation. The contribution of a pharmacist or other member of the pain management team is essential to working toward pain control because it can be especially complex in the presence of obesity (Box 2).

Box 2. Understanding the resedation phenomenon

Resedation is a postoperative threat among larger patients. Davidson and Callery [20] explain that by the evening of surgery, the overt effects of intraoperative anesthesia have dissipated. The patient may be using postoperative pain medication, but this is the time when the patient is most prone to the resedation phenomenon. Resedation occurs when the redistribution of lipophilic anesthetic or sedative agents from the fatty tissue enters the bloodstream. The challenge of resedation is that pharmacologic reversal or intubation may be urgently necessary, which poses a life-threatening situation if not managed in a timely manner.

The Wound Ostomy Continence Nurse offers a plan of care to address the local abdominal wound care, which typically occurs among obese patients undergoing panniculectomy. The entire health care team must be diligent in caring for the morbidly obese patient. Being aware of the possible complications and corresponding interventions is necessary to prevent potential hazards to patient and caregivers. Communication and timing are critical to prevent these hazards. Although it is sometimes difficult to arrange, an interdisciplinary conference, which is planned within 24 hours of admission, may prevent costly intervention from occurring later [19]. Consider including the patient's significant other because this person may offer insight into the patient's special needs. Documentation of meetings, individual goals, and corresponding intervention promote consistent, meaningful patient care and may protect the institution from legal action. This level of accountability also outlines more fully each clinician's responsibilities.

Preparing for the future

Although attempts to reduce body weight are common among Americans, the prevalence of obesity continues to increase. Considering that more than two thirds of US adults are overweight, it is likely that issues of caring for the overweight patient will continue. In fact, not only has the percentage of adult American increased but the number of overweight children has doubled, and although some overweight people are able to lose some of their body weight, a majority regains that weight within 5 years.

Such increases will tremendously affect health care delivery because obesity is strongly associated with several chronic diseases, which may lead to hospitalization and the corresponding issues described earlier. Recent estimates suggest that obesity-related morbidity may account for 6.8% of

---

Box 3. Planning for equipment

Patients who weigh more than 300 pounds generally require
some level of special accommodation. In many cases, the
only special accommodation that is needed is a bed that is
wide enough for the patient to turn independently, a walker
to support their weight, and an overhead trapeze to help
the patient reposition him or herself. These three items
are believed to help the patient maintain strength and
independence. Clinicians report that independent patients
who have adequate supportive equipment are less likely to
injure themselves or caregivers during that early
postoperative period [22].

US health care costs. This increasing prevalence will affect acute care and
may influence not only the frequency of admission but the intensity of care
that patients will require when hospitalized. Clinicians best serve the needs
of the patient when policies and protocols are in place to care for the
patient. Continued use of interdisciplinary teams is essential to more fully
understand the interdepartmental impact of caring for overweight patients
in the acute care setting. Furthermore, manufacturers and vendors need
clinical input to more fully understand the unique equipment needs of the
larger patient (Box 3). Clinicians can form partnerships with industry to
creatively seek solutions to the challenges described, and outcome studies
can provide the data necessary to sustain these efforts.

Summary

With obesity on the rise, clinicians must use strategies to reduce or
prevent costly complications. Although equipment is a helpful adjunct to
care, it is never a substitute for care. Numerous resources are available to
clinicians across practice settings, and the use of resources in a timely and
appropriate manner is believed to improve measurable therapeutic,
satisfaction, and cost outcomes. Unquestionably, clinicians and organizations are continually at risk for legal action, but there are steps that can be
taken to control for meritless claims. The obese patient poses numerous care
challenges, and it is in the interest of health care organizations to meet these
challenges in a clinically and legally sound manner.

References

[1] Kral JG, Strauss RJ, Wise L. Perioperative risk management in obese patients. In: Deitl M,
    editor. Surgery for the morbidly obese patient. North York: FD Communications; 2000.
    p. 238–61.

[2] Gallagher S. Meeting the needs of the obese patient. Am J Nurs 1996;96(8):1s–12s.
[3] Gallagher S. Taking the weight off with bariatric surgery. Nursing 2004;34(3):58–64.
[4] Frontline fat PBS home video. Seattle (WA): Public Broadcasting Service; 1998.
[5] Fox HR. Discrimination: alive and well in the United States. Obes Surg 1995;5:21.
[6] Kuczmarski RJ, Fiegel KM, Campbell SM, et al. Increasing prevalence of overweight among US adults: the national health and nutrition examination surveys, 1960 to 1991. JAMA 1994; 272:205–11.
[7] Gustafson NJ. Managing obesity and eating disorders. Brockton (MA): Western Schools Press; 1997. p. 2.
[8] Staffieri JR. A study of social stereotype of body image in children. J Pers Soc Psychol 1967;7: 101–4.
[9] Thone RR. Fat: a fate worse than death. New York: Harrington Park Press; 1997.
[10] Maiman LA, Wang VL, Becker MH, et al. Attitudes toward obesity and the obese among professionals. J Am Diet Assoc 1992;74:331–6.
[11] Gallagher SM. Morbid obesity: a chronic disease with an impact on wounds and related problems. Ostomy Wound Manage 1997;43(5):18–27.
[12] Gustafson NJ. Managing obesity and eating disorders. Toronto, Canada: Western Schools Press; 1997. p. 13–19.
[13] Gallagher SM. Caring for obese patients. Nursing 1998;98(3):32HN1–32HN5.
[14] Troia C. The obese patient. Plast Surg Nurs 2002;22(1):10–8.
[15] Gallagher S. Panniculectomy, documentation, reimbursement and the WOC nurse. J Wound Ostomy Continence Nurs 2003;30(2):72–7.
[16] Cowan SM, Wallace RD, Marx A, et al. Plastic surgery after loss of massive excess weight. In: Dietel M, Cowan SM, editors. Update: surgery for the morbidly obese patient. Toronto: FD Communications; 2000. p. 262–91.
[17] Gallagher SM. Tailoring care for the obese patient. RN 1999;62(5):43–50.
[18] Freiberg A. Plastic surgery after massive weight loss. In: Dietel M, editor. Surgery for the morbidly obese patient. Toronto: FD Communications; 1998.
[19] DeRuiter HP, Meitteunen E, Sauder K. Improving safety for caregivers through collaborative practice. Journal of Healthcare Safety, Compliance, and Infection Control 2001;5(2):61–4.
[20] Davidson J, Callery C. Care of the obesity surgery patient requiring immediate-level care or intensive care. Obes Surg 2001;11:93–7.
[21] Lindstrom W. So you want your insurance to cover your obesity surgery? Center for Law and Advocacy. Available at: http://www.obesitylaw.com/insurancearticle.htm. Accessed April 1, 2004.
[22] Gallagher SM. Restructuring the therapeutic environment to promote care and safety for obese patient. J Wound Ostomy Continence Nurs 1999;26:292–7.

NURSING
CLINICS
OF NORTH AMERICA

Nurs Clin N Am 40 (2005) 337–347

Spinal Cord Injury and Pressure Ulcers

Maria Helena Larcher Caliri, PhD, RN

*Ribeirao Preto School of Nursing, University of Sao Paulo, Av. Bandeirantes, 3900 Ribeirao
Preto, Sao Paulo, 14040-902-Brazil*

Spinal cord injury (SCI) is often cited as one of most devastating type of
injury because it instantly creates lifelong physiologic, emotional, social, and
economic alteration to the person and the family [1]. Until World War II, the
health care philosophy for the SCI patient was that it was not advantageous
to invest energy and time to treat them because negative outcomes could be
anticipated. As a consequence of medical complications such as urinary tract
infection, pressure ulcers, and sepsis, life expectancy was short. After World
War II, countries were faced with large numbers of people with injuries
involving the central nervous system. Rehabilitation programs specifically
for SCI were developed in Great Britain and the United States.

In the 1970s in the United States, a new philosophy of care emerged,
which culminated with the establishment of regional spinal cord injury
centers, later designated as the Model Spinal Cord Injury System. Services
required by the patient from the time of injury and throughout life were
provided, including appropriate medical and surgical care, health maintenance, and crisis intervention. Even with the advances in health care and new
technologies, the person with a SCI is at risk for pressure ulcer development.
A pressure ulcer is seen as a frequent, costly, and life-threatening condition
that results in long hospitalization and interferes with rehabilitation and
community reintegration.

Pressure ulcer statistics

According to the 1998 National Spinal Cord Injury Statistical Center
Annual Report [2], 34% of individuals admitted to a Model Systems facility
within 24 hours of SCI developed at least one pressure ulcer during acute care
or rehabilitation. McKinley et al [3] identified pressure ulcers as the most
common secondary complication in all years after injury; an increased

E-mail address: mhcaliri@eerp.usp.br

prevalence was associated with greater number of years after injury. The National Pressure Ulcer Advisory Panel [4] indicated that the incidence of pressure ulcers ranged between 20% for those undergoing spinal surgery and 31% 1 year after the injury. Prevalence rates ranged from 10.2% to 30% at the first annual examination. Early studies [5] estimated that in the United States between 50% and 80% of persons with SCI developed a pressure ulcer at least once in their lives. The majority of the ulcers occurred in the first 2 years after injury, but even after 3 to 4 years, there was a reported incidence of 30%.

Pressure ulcer statistics have been examined worldwide. In the United Kingdom, 32% of patients arrived at a spinal cord injury unit with pressure ulcers, whereas a total of 56% experienced an ulcer at some stage between injury and discharge [6]. Pressure ulcers were associated with an increased length of hospital stay, complete lesion (American Spinal Injury Association, grade A), surgical stabilization of neck injury before transfer to the spinal cord unit, tracheostomy on admission, and delayed transfer to the SCI unit after injury. Noreau et al [7] in Quebec reported the prevalence of secondary impairments among individuals with long-standing SCI as urinary tract infection (56%), spasticity (40%), hypotension (33%), autonomic dysreflexia (31%) and pressure ulcers (28%). A Brazilian survey [8] of patients with SCI revealed 54% had pressure ulcers. Comparing statistics about SCI for different countries is difficult because of varying methodology used for data collection, the social, political, economic and sanitary levels of the country, and the environmental aspects.

The cost of pressure ulcers in the SCI population is difficult to obtain. In the United States, health care costs associated with SCI are estimated to be $1.5 to $2 million over the lifetime of a person [9]. After the initial medical care and rehabilitation, the majority of these costs are associated with complications and hospital readmissions for secondary impairments, including pressure ulcers [9]. Recurrence of pressure ulcers after healing has been reported as high as 35% for patients with SCI. However, pressure ulcers impact multiple aspects of function, thus there are personal costs that interfere with the rehabilitation process and are a significant deterrent to activities that contribute to independent, productive, and satisfying lives. For both the individual and the caregiver, pressure ulcers can result in time missed from work or school, delayed community reintegration, reduced quality of life, and loss of self-esteem [2].

Evidence-based practice recommendations

It is imperative that SCI individuals develop effective strategies for self-management of skin care. They need guidance and assistance in the decisions required to restore health, independent function, and self-esteem, as well as ways to prevent and treat pressure ulcers, if they occur. The Consortium for Spinal Cord Medicine developed the guideline Pressure Ulcer Prevention and

Treatment Following Spinal Cord Injury [2] as part of a series of evidence-based clinical practice documents to provide the conceptual framework within which effective strategies for preventing and treating pressure ulcers could be developed. The recommendations of the guideline are based on an extensive review and analysis of the available scientific literature and represent the most current understanding of interventions applied in clinical practice. The scientific level of research was based hierarchically with the greatest weight placed on randomized, controlled trials followed by obser-vational studies, uncontrolled case series, and case reports. When evidence from the literature was lacking, the recommendations were based on expert opinion. Every recommendation was assessed by considering the level of agreement of the members of the panel.

Most of the recommendations proposed in the SCI guideline are the same as those presented in the Clinical Practice Guidelines related to pressure ulcer in adults, developed by the Agency for Healthcare Research and Quality (formerly the Agency for Health Care Policy and Research). However, Pressure Ulcer Prevention and Treatment Following Spinal Cord Injury emphasizes the characteristics of the SCI population that make them prone to pressure ulcers and conditions that aggravate the risk. Box 1 summarizes the preventive care strategies from this document.

Pressure ulcer risk

Pressure ulcer risk in SCI people is a complex problem that transcends the biomechanical aspects of the soft tissue response to mechanical loading. Health care professionals and researchers must look beyond the obvious issues of risk and focus on the patient's intrinsic and extrinsic characteristics that influence the pressure ulcer formation. Assessment scales are seen as tools that can heighten the health care professional's awareness of which patients need more aggressive pressure ulcer preventive measures [10]. Most individuals with SCI will be at risk for pressure ulcers according to general scales such as the Braden scale as well as the scale for persons with paralysis [11]. Research is needed to establish the predictive merit for SCI risk assessment variables.

Individuals with SCI have neurologically impaired skin. Interference of the catabolism and biosynthesis of collagen of the skin may decrease the elasticity of skin. The skin is less able to adapt to mechanical insult. Tensile strength is decreased, producing a more fragile skin below the level of injury. All individuals with SCI should be considered as high risk for pressure ulcers in all settings and receive effective preventive strategies. Conditions that are seen as increasing the risk are aging and presence of comorbidities, longer duration of SCI, level and completeness of injury, and level of activity and mobility [2]. Other factors associated with increased risk are history of previous pressure ulcers, surgical repair of pressure ulcers, belief in the susceptibility to pressure ulcers, younger age at onset of SCI, more

---

Box 1. Summary of the Preventive Care in the Pressure Ulcer Prevention and Treatment Following Spinal Cord Injury report

1. Conduct systematic and consistent assessment of pressure ulcer risk factors of individuals with SCI
2. Implement prevention strategies as part of the comprehensive management of acute SCI
3. Conduct daily comprehensive visual and tactile skin inspection with particular attention to the areas most vulnerable to pressure ulcer development
4. Turn or reposition individuals with SCI initially every 2 hours in the acute and rehabilitation phases if the medical condition allows
5. Evaluate the individual and his or her support environment for optimal maintenance of skin integrity
6. Provide an individually prescribed wheel chair and pressure-reducing seating system
7. Implement an ongoing exercise regimen for the medically stable individual to promote maintenance of skin integrity, increase strength of muscles, improve cardiovascular endurance, and prevent fatigue and deconditioning
8. Provide individuals with SCI, their families, significant others, and health-care professionals with specific information on effective strategies for the prevention and treatment of pressure ulcers
9. Assess the nutritional status of all SCI individuals on admission and as needed, based on medical status
10. Provide adequate nutritional intake to meet the individual's needs
11. Implement aggressive nutritional support measures if dietary intake is inadequate or if an individual is nutritionally compromised

---

years of smoking, and delay in seeking treatment or taking preventive measures [12]. Regular skin assessments should be incorporated into the patient's overall comprehensive assessment.

There are limited studies relating the association of risk with psychologic and social factors. If the person has psychologic distress, cognitive impairment, or is in a situation of substance abuse, adherence to health recommendations has the potential to be compromised. Krause [13] examined the relationship between pressure ulcers and life adjustment after traumatic SCI. Persons with pressure ulcers had lower levels of subjective well being and activity as well as greater health problems compared with those without pressure ulcers. The number of days of having a pressure ulcer, the number of wounds, and the inability to tolerate sitting because of pressure ulcers were strong risk factors for poorer scores on life adjustment indices [13].

Pressure ulcer prevention and management

The activities involved in managing SCI are complex and involve life changes. Many of the interventions that are necessary for pressure ulcer prevention require understanding, cooperation, and initiative on the part of the individual who has the injury or from those that do the formal or informal care. Preventive care might be compromised by the lack of social or financial support [2]. Strategies for the prevention of pressure ulcers require management of mechanical forces such as turning, weight shifts while seated, chair cushions, and other devices [12,14,15]. SCI individuals have a life-long need to use pressure-reducing support surfaces that are effective in reducing interface pressures. Evaluation of support surfaces for the bed and chair must be considered in terms of pressure readings over time, durability, cost, and comfort, among other factors. Seating evaluation should be available as part of continuum of care. Poor equipment conditions will contribute to the development of a pressure ulcer or retard its healing [2].

Incontinence and moisture are factors associated with pressure ulcers because of the neurogenic bowel and bladder condition that occurs with SCI [11]. To reduce the risk, incontinence needs to be assessed and managed [12]. Recommendations related to the management of incontinence include the establishment of a bowel and bladder program, selection of an incontinence skin barrier, and the collection, containment, or wicking of incontinence away from the skin [12].

Nutrition is a critical component of pressure ulcer prevention and care. A hypermetabolic, potentially catabolic state occurs in SCI patients with pressure ulcers [16]. Measuring an SCI person's energy expenditure to determine caloric requirements has been strongly recommended to achieve better treatment results [16]. Nonhealing wounds are associated with malnutrition, smoking, intercurrent illnesses, substance abuse, and the absence of social support [17]. Successful healing of pressure ulcers is associated with adequate wound management, pressure reduction, maintenance of an optimal nutritional status, and patient education and adherence to preventive measures.

If a pressure ulcer develops, wound assessment should be comprehensive. An objective and thorough description of the wound enables the development of an appropriate treatment plan, forms the basis for serial assessment to determine outcomes, and provides a reliable means of communicating wound status among health professionals [2]. The assessment of posture, positioning, and equipment is critical in determining the cause of the wound and the development of treatment strategies. Wound care should follow general recommendations for chronic wounds [18]. Individuals with stage III and IV pressure ulcers that do not respond to conservative wound therapy may need surgical repair. Successful postoperative management depends on modifying the factors that contributed to the ulcer formation and teaching "pressure consciousness" to the individual [2].

Education of the patient

A gap exists in the evaluation of educational programs to promote adherence to the preventive behaviors necessary to reduce the occurrence or recurrence of pressure ulcers, especially after the person has returned home [2]. Nursing practice emphasizes the importance of patient and family education for health promotion. Studies are necessary to test interventions that enhance the achievement of rehabilitation outcomes, facilitate knowledge acquisition and decision making, reduce complications and cost associated with SCI, and contribute to the quality of life for individuals and caregivers [9]. A predictor of adherence to healthy behaviors, such as the prevention of pressure ulcers, is the relationship and communication between the person and those making recommendations for care [2]. Individuals often do not understand or retain health behavior instructions the first time such instructions are given. The person's ability to verbalize the prescribed health behavior regimen is a minimum indicator of adherence [2].

Education to prevent pressure ulcers should include multiple factors. Information must be accurate and consistent. The person should be taught to make decisions or alter behavior when life circumstances change and to anticipate situations that may hinder skin care. Written information may be used to complement verbal explanations. The literacy level of the patient and family must be considered when selecting written materials. Yasenchak and Bridle [19] developed and evaluated an educational module about pressure ulcers for persons with low literacy skills. With this manual, knowledge scores increased before and after testing and were maintained after discharge. Alternatives to printed materials such as audiotapes, videotapes, and demonstrations need to be used to complement educational programs for individuals who have low literacy or when the primary language is not English. Viehbeck et al [20] showed the effectiveness of a videotape to teach the adverse effects of cigarette smoking on pressure ulcer prevention and healing.

A person's life style may affect learning. Every person presents a unique existence that reflects a network of psychologic traits, goals, values, preferred activities, environmental opportunities and challenges, habits, routines, and personal practices [21]. Embedded in this context of daily activities and concerns is the distinct pattern of risk for pressure ulcers for each individual. Krause et al [22] noted that the primary protective behaviors for pressure ulcers were general characteristics (ie, employment, marital status, and years of education) rather than specific health maintenance or promotion behaviors. The examination of daily activities allows an understanding of pressure ulcer risk and contributes to the patient's lifestyle redesign to reduce the occurrence of ulcers. Educational programs that promote an overall healthy style may be more successful in reducing risk for pressure ulcers than those specifically aimed at skin care.

Because most education programs for pressure ulcer prevention are designed for the initial hospitalization and rehabilitation, outpatient educational programs are greatly needed to reinforce pressure ulcer detection and treatment. More emphasis needs to be placed on patients' responsibilities for the prevention and management of pressure ulcers after discharge. Patients who developed pressure ulcers at home and took immediate action reported an average of 3.6 preventive behaviors, whereas patients who delayed action until the next day had an average of 2.4 preventive behaviors [23]. Patients who waited longer to come to the clinic had ulcers that progressed to a greater severity and showed less ability to accurately describe their ulcer [23]. The perceived severity of a pressure ulcer, the perceived efficacy of skin care, and an individual's beliefs have been positively correlated with compliance with skin care [24]. SCI people often lack the necessary long-term knowledge or resources to deal with pressure ulcers.

The time for professional contact with patients has decreased because of the shorter length of stay and the introduction of unlicensed personnel to assist with patient care [9]. Following discharge from rehabilitation centers, persons with SCI are at a greater risk for pressure ulcers because when they attempt to be independent, are employed, or are involved with education, they may neglect to follow even the most basic skin care regimen taught to them during hospitalization [5]. Nurses and therapists contribute to the achievement of rehabilitation outcomes using every interaction with clients as an opportunity to share information, provide support, or address questions and concerns. As the time for patient and family education decreases, it is necessary to identify the most effective means of achieving desired patient outcomes.

Compliance with care

Interventions need to include strategies that establish positive consequences for engaging in effective pressure ulcer prevention behaviors. Traditional nursing and educational approaches to pressure ulcer prevention may not be effective with patients who have recurrent ulcers. Recurrence may be unavoidable in some cases because of factors beyond the individual's control (eg, increased susceptibility after successive wounds). For other patients, pressure ulcers develop because of persistent noncompliance with recommended preventive strategies.

Jones et al [25] examined a three-part intervention strategy for SCI persons, which consists of a mutually developed provider-patient health plan, a graduated schedule of outpatient clinic visits, and financial rewards for remaining pressure ulcer free. The authors concluded that this approach may be effective among individuals with high recidivism. The money given to participants may have been used to improve their living conditions, such as to purchase food, obtain needed supplies, or pay for personal assistance, thus subsequently contributing to better skin care. It is necessary to determine whether contingent reinforcement is necessary or if simply providing better follow-up care and more resources alone would lead to greater success.

Nurses are in a position to help patients identify the problems and behavioral changes that are necessary for long-term care. Because a patient's readiness to change is critical in achieving successful outcomes, the nurse can use various theoretical models to help patients with change. For example, the Transtheorethical Model of Readiness for Change [26] helps to identify mutually accepted goals and to determine the best way to help the patient assume self-care responsibilities. The model stipulates that changing from high-risk behavior to behavior that enhances health promotion requires following five stages of change: (1) precontemplation, when there is no intent to change; (2) contemplation, when there is thought for change; (3) preparation, when serious consideration for change develops; (4) action, when the individual is actively changing his or her behavior; and (5) maintenance, when the individual is sustaining the changed behavior for 6 months or more.

Telerehabilitation

Comprehensive rehabilitation centers for SCI provide an environment in which patients and families can gain confidence in self-care skills and adjust psychologically to the catastrophic injury. In a managed care environment, inpatient lengths of stay have been greatly reduced, affecting the patient's ability to integrate preventive behaviors into daily life. Yet those behaviors are essential for avoiding serious health problems and common complications. The challenge to clinician is to find cost-effective ways to extend the continuum of care into the home and community-based settings so that functional outcomes do not suffer. Pressure ulcers, if present, require frequent assessment to ensure that treatment is appropriate and effective. The SCI person may be challenged to find transportation and keep frequent outpatient visits. Because of advances in technology, a mobile unit with simultaneous transmission of video and audio data connected to the patient's home television can be used to send images back and forth from clinician to patient during conversation [27]. At the health care institution, a computer can be used to store and print the images. In testing the process, Vesmarovich et al [27] noted that pressure ulcer management was performed successfully by "telerehabilitation." An unexpected advantage of seeing the patient in the home was the visualization of the home environment and the patient and family's behaviors that many times deter the wound from healing. Telerehabilitation facilitated earlier intervention and prevention of wound deterioration.

Education of health professionals and nurses' roles

Professionals who work with SCI struggle to provide quality care to improve patients' lives in the absence of good evidence to guide their treatment decisions. SCI patients often develop other problems such as urinary tract infection and pneumonia and are rehospitalized. While investigating patterns of service delivery for the management of pressure ulcers for the SCI and their families, Wellard and Rushton [28] identified the environment in which the care was delivered as a central factor. Nogueira et al [29] studied professional and ancillary nurses' perceptions of causes of pressure ulcers and preventive measures for SCI individuals. The process and structure of care within the institution did not focus on prevention; turning of the patient was not rigorously carried out, and bed mattresses were inadequate, resulting in an excess of pressure on bone prominences. The care of pressure ulcers was less valued than other clinical problems. The focus of attention was more on medical problems instead of the prevention of pressure ulcers. The patient arrived at the health care setting with one problem but may have left with more problems because the process and structure of care were lacking. Beliefs about the importance of preventive care varied across the level of the nurses' education, with the most highly educated nurses identifying prevention as the most important. Continued education of all levels of nursing providers is necessary [29].

Guihan et al [30] examined the variability in clinical decisions made by health care professionals about pressure ulcer management for the SCI population. The availability of social support was the most important factor in deciding whether the patient was managed at home or in the hospital rather than the level of spinal cord injury. For patients with poor social support, more healing was required before discharge, regardless of medical condition. The health professionals agreed that patients who were compliant with prevention measures could avoid ulcer development.

The World Health Organization emphasizes that nurses have a vital function in health promotion and prevention of health problems in rehabilitation [31]. In developed countries, the majority of people with disabling conditions has the opportunity to receive rehabilitation and specialized services. In developing countries, only 15% of persons in urban areas and 2% of persons in rural regions receive these services. The World Health Organization proposes that in countries where services are deficient care be provided through the Universal Health System using resources that are available within the community, and nurses should be educated to work within this system [31].

In North America, pressure ulcers have received the attention of governments, regulatory agencies, lawyers, and health benefit payers because of the enormous economic burden [32]. Programs must be developed that go across the care continuum, including the community using evidence-based guidelines to promote best practice.

Summary

The SCI person is at high risk for pressure ulcers; thus, pressure ulcer prevention is a critical component of care. Guidelines exist to promote evidenced-based practice for the prevention and treatment of pressure ulcers in the SCI. There is a discrepancy between what persons with SCI know about pressure ulcer prevention and what they are doing to reduce their risk of developing this serious complication. Objective data demonstrate that adherence to a skin care regimen contributes to the prevention of pressure ulcers. Knowledge about pressure ulcer prevention and treatment must be appropriately focused for the patient, family, and the health care team and must be reinforced over time.

References

[1] Metcalf JA. Acute phase management of persons with spinal cord injury: a nursing diagnosis perspective. Nurs Clin North Am 1986;21(4):589–98.

[2] Paralyzed Veterans of America. Pressure ulcer prevention and treatment following spinal cord injury: a clinical practice guideline for health-care professionals. Washington (DC): Paralyzed Veterans of America; 2000. p. 1–94.

[3] McKinley WO, Jackson AB, Cardenas DD, et al. Long term medical complications after traumatic spinal cord injury: a regional model systems analysis. Arch Phys Med Rehabil 1999;80:1402–10.

[4] Cuddigan J, Sprigle S, Brienza D. Pressure ulcers in persons with spinal cord injuries. In: Cuddigan J, Ayello EA, Sussman C, editors. Pressure ulcers in America: prevalence, incidence and implications for the future. Reston (VA): National Pressure Ulcer Advisory Panel; 2001. p. 129–31.

[5] Rodrigues GP, Garber SL. Prospective study of pressure ulcer risk in spinal cord injury patients. Paraplegia 1994;32:150–8.

[6] Ash D. An exploration of the occurrence of pressure ulcers in a British spinal injuries unit. J Clin Nurs 2002;11(4):470–8.

[7] Noreau L, Proulx P, Gagnon L, et al. Secondary impairments after spinal cord injury: a population-based study. Am J Phys Med Rehabil 2000;79(6):526–35.

[8] Da Paz AC, Beraldo PS, Almeida MC, et al. Traumatic injury to the spinal cord: prevalence in Brazilian hospitals. Paraplegia 1992;30(9):636–40.

[9] Lucke KT. Outcomes of nurse caring as perceived by individuals with spinal cord injury during rehabilitation. Rehabil Nurs 1999;24(6):247–53.

[10] Bergstrom N, Braden B, Boynton P, et al. Using a research-based assessment scale in clinical practice. Nurs Clin North Am 1995;30(3):539–51.

[11] Salzberg CA, Byrne DW, Cayten CG, et al. Predicting and preventing pressure ulcers in adults with paralysis. Adv Wound Care 1998;11(5):237–46.

[12] Wound Ostomy Continence Nurses Society (WOCN). Guideline for prevention and management of pressure ulcers. WOCN Clinical Practice Guidelines series. Glenview (IL): WOCN; 2003. p. 5.

[13] Krause JS. Skin sores after spinal cord injury: relationship to life adjustment. Spinal Cord 1998;36(5):1–56.

[14] Bergstrom N, Allman RM, Carlson CR, et al. Pressure ulcers in adults: prediction and prevention. Clinical Practice Guideline. number 3. Rockville, MD, Agency for Health Care Policy and Research; 1992. US Department of Health and Human Services. AHCPR Publication #92–0047.

[15] Pieper B. Mechanical forces: pressure, shear, and friction. In: Bryant RA, editor. Acute and chronic wounds: nursing management. 2nd edition. St. Louis (MO): Mosby; 2000. p. 221–64.

[16] Liu MH, Spungen AM, Fink L, et al. Increased energy needs in patients with quadriplegia and pressure ulcers. Adv Wound Care 1996;9(3):41–5.

[17] Niazi ZBM, Salzberg CA, Byrne DW, et al. Recurrence of initial pressure ulcer in persons with spinal cord injuries. Adv Wound Care 1997;10(3):38–42.

[18] Krasner DL, Sibbald RG. Nursing management of chronic wounds: best practices across the continuum of care. Nurs Clin North Am 1999;34(4):933–53.

[19] Yasenchak PA, Bridle MJ. A low-literacy skin care manual for spinal cord injury patients. Patient Educ Couns 1993;22:1–5.

[20] Viehbeck M, McGlynn J, Harris S. Pressure ulcers and wound healing: educating the spinal cord injured individual on the effects of cigarette smoking. SCI Nurs 1995;12(3):73–6.

[21] Clark F, Rubayi S, Jackson J, et al. The role of daily activities in pressure ulcer development. Adv Skin Wound Care 2001;14(2):52–4.

[22] Krause JS, Vines CL, Farley TL, et al. An exploratory study of pressure ulcers after spinal cord injury: relationship to protective behaviors and risk factors. Arch Phys Rehabil 2001; 82(1):107–13.

[23] Garber SL, Rintala DH, Rossi CD, et al. Reported pressure ulcer prevention and management techniques by persons with spinal cord injury. Arch Phys Med Rehabil 1996; 77(8):744–9.

[24] Dai Y, Catanzaro M. Health beliefs and compliance with a skin care regimen. Rehabil Nurs 1987;12(1):13–6.

[25] Jones ML, Mathewson CS, Adkins VK, et al. Use of behavioral contingencies to promote prevention of reccurrent pressure ulcers. Arch Phys Med Rehabil 2003;84(6):796–802.

[26] Rivera E, Walsh A, Bradley M. Using behavior modifications to promote wound healing. Home Healthc Nurse 2000;18(9):579–86.

[27] Vesmarovich S, Walker T, Hauber RP, et al. Use of telerehabilitation to manage pressure ulcers in persons with spinal cord injuries. Adv Wound Care 1999;12(5):264–9.

[28] Wellard S, Rushton C. Influences of spatial practices on pressure ulcer management in the context of spinal cord injury. Int J Nurs Pract 2002;8(4):221–7.

[29] Nogueira PC, Caliri MH, Santos CB. Risk factors and prevention of pressure ulcer in spinal cord injury patients: experience of members of nursing team at FMRP-USP Hospital. Medicina (Ribeirao Preto) 2002;35(1):14–23.

[30] Guihan M, Goldstein B, Schwartz A, et al. SCI health care provider attitudes about pressure ulcer management. J Spinal Cord Med 2003;26(2):129–34.

[31] World Health Organization. Disability prevention and rehabilitation: a guide for strengthening the basic nursing curriculum. Rehabilitation Unit. Division of Health Promotion, Education, and Communication, WHO, 1996. Available at: http://www.who.int/ncd/disability/publications.htm. Accessed February 20, 2004.

[32] Junkin J. Promoting healthy skin in various settings. Nurs Clin North Am 2000;35(2): 339–48.

ELSEVIER
SAUNDERS

Nurs Clin N Am 40 (2005) 349–363

NURSING
CLINICS
OF NORTH AMERICA

Injection Drug Use and Wound Care

Barbara Pieper, PhD, RN, CS, CWOCN, FAAN[a,b,*],
John A. Hopper, MD[c]

[a]College of Nursing, Wayne State University, 5557 Cass Avenue, Detroit, MI 48202, USA
[b]Detroit Receiving Hospital, Detroit, MI 48202, USA
[c]School of Medicine, Wayne State University, 2761 East Jefferson, Detroit,
MI 48207, USA

Substance abuse is considered a major health problem in the United States, with 22.3% of deaths attributed to alcohol, tobacco, and illicit drug use [1]. The use of injection drugs accounts for 12% of all illicit drug use in the United States [2]. Three main routes of injection are recognized: intravenous, subcutaneous, and intramuscular. The term "injection drug use" encompasses all three routes. The drug most commonly injected is heroin; at least 3 million Americans over the age of 12 have used heroin at least once in their lifetime [3]. Injection drug use is found in men and women and in all educational levels. It tends to be more of an urban problem and affects disproportionate numbers of minority persons. Injection drug users fit many profiles, ranging from those who injected drugs for a short time and quit to those who inject for their entire lives. Some stop injecting drugs but continue to use illicit drugs by other routes such as smoking or inhaling. There is wide diversity in a person's drug history and in the types of wounds that may be seen. This article focuses on two types of wounds, wounds after drainage of an abscess and venous ulcers, and care considerations.

Injection drug classes and consequences

The major injection drugs of abuse in North America are opiates, including heroin, and stimulants such as cocaine and methamphetamine. Injection of sedatives such as barbiturates and benzodiazepines is much less common. Different classes of drugs have different patterns of use and may result in different consequences. Regardless of the "drug of choice," most

---

* Corresponding author. College of Nursing, Wayne State University, 5557 Cass Avenue, Detroit, MI 48202.

E-mail address: bpieper@wayne.edu (B. Pieper).

0029-6465/05/$ - see front matter © 2005 Elsevier Inc. All rights reserved.
doi:10.1016/j.cnur.2004.09.010
nursing.theclinics.com

injection drug users are "polysubstance" abusers [4]. Among drug injectors, tobacco dependence is high, and the use of marijuana and alcohol is also greater than in the general population. Combined drug use probably leads to greater consequences from injecting, such as impaired wound healing among chronic tobacco smokers. All drug injection increases the risk of acute infections (eg, abscesses), and long-term intravenous injection may lead to chronic venous insufficiency and, ultimately, to venous ulcers.

Heroin and cocaine

Heroin is the prototypical opiate analgesic and produces euphoria, noted as a feeling of relaxation, sedation, and calm, and freedom from worry and pain. After the "high" from heroin, the person experiences irritability, despair, anxiety, decreased sedation, and increased pain. Tolerance to the euphoria develops, resulting in the person increasing the amount of the drug used. Heroin withdrawal typically occurs 3 to 5 hours after the last use, with manifestations of craving, anxiety, sleep disturbances, muscle spasms, joint pain, tremor, tachycardia, hypertension, and abdominal cramps, to name a few side effects. Heroin use has many patterns. Some persons experiment with heroin and only use it a few times; others use it occasionally, and this is referred to as "chipping." Regular or daily use may evolve over time, with most dependent persons injecting three to six times per day [5]. Polysubstance abuse among heroin users may show specific patterns of drug use. Tobacco and cocaine may be used to moderate the depressive effect; alcohol and other sedatives are used to moderate withdrawal symptoms, to enhance the opiate high, and to act as a substitute when heroin is not available [6].

Cocaine is classified as an indirect sympathetic agonist. As a psychostimulant, it causes euphoria, hyperactive behavior, irritability, restlessness, disturbed sleep, anorexia, attention difficulty, and perceptions of increased strength and sexual function. It is a powerful vasoconstrictor that results in marked cardiovascular changes such as increased blood pressure, cardiac arrhythmia, and angina. Withdrawal from cocaine use results in an intense craving for more of the drug, depression, apathy, and lethargy. Cocaine can be inhaled, injected, or absorbed through any mucous membrane. When cocaine is injected with heroin, it is referred to as "speedballing."

Injection process

The preferred site of drug injection is the intravenous route ("mainlining") because of the fast response of the drug. If the vein is missed or there is too much venous destruction, the drug may be injected subcutaneously ("skin popping") or intramuscularly ("muscling"). An artery may be hit accidentally or intentionally, causing a burning sensation, paresthesia, and hyperemic flush over the arterial distribution. Spasm of the artery and subsequent ischemia may develop. Injecting drugs can occur within a person's own environment or with others in a "shooting gallery." The person may inject him- or herself or have it injected by someone else. Thus, there is a high probability of sharing drug equipment, thereby increasing the risk of spread of disease.

The substances injected and the injection process lead to many of the infection and wound problems for injection drug users. The drug is sold after it has been diluted or "cut" with other substances. These substances are often fillers; and the person does not know the amount of drug purchased or what the fillers are. The most common filler is quinine because it is similar in appearance and taste to heroin. Fillers may cause vasospasm, intimal damage, thrombus, and particulate embolization. To prepare the drug for injection, it may be diluted with water from any source, cooked over a flame to liquefy, and filtered with a piece of cotton or cigarette filter placed in it and around the needle. Saliva is often used to lubricate the needle or moisten the cotton filter. Tablets may be crushed between the teeth. Using the mouth, clots of blood and other particulate matter are blown from the injection paraphernalia. Injection equipment ("works") may be used many times and shared with others, thus increasing contamination. Drug injectors often do not clean the injection site before injecting. The nature of the injection process may also influence the likelihood of developing infection. Intramuscular and subcutaneous injections appear to be more commonly associated with skin infection compared with intravenous injections [7,8].

Abscess and infection

Abscess formation at the site of drug injection is the most common infectious complication of injection drug use [9]. Cellulitis is frequently present with an abscess. Skin and soft tissue infections are a common reason for hospitalization for persons who inject drugs [10]. The mechanism for establishing infection probably relates to tissue trauma, direct effect of the drugs, tissue ischemia, and inoculation of bacteria [11]. Repeated injection damages the skin and tissue. The drugs, especially cocaine, may cause vasospasm and thrombosis. Immune disorders may contribute to the person's predisposition to infection. Opiates may suppress several T-cell functions that are important for cell-mediated immunity and also inhibit phagocytosis, chemotaxis, and filling of polymorphonuclear neutrophil leukocytes and macrophage [11]. Localized deposition of injected substances, as with subcutaneous and intramuscular injections, provides a focus for infection, whereas drugs that are injected intravenously are rapidly dispersed [12].

A person with an abscess will often present with a localized site of infection. Bergstein et al [9] identified the most common presenting signs and symptoms of abscess as pain and tenderness (100%), erythema (93%), fluctuance (74%), leukocytosis (54%), lymphadenopathy (48%), and fever (42%). Sometimes infections are deeper in the muscle and fascia and will not present with typical manifestations. These deeper sites may spread to adjacent tissues and cause local swelling, leading to obstruction of organs and tissues, and cause osteomyelitis, arterial pseudoaneurysm, and compartment syndrome [11,13,14]. Cultures are best taken from the fluid that is aspirated or drained from the site. The most common aerobes are *Staphylococcus aureus* and *Streptococcus* spp [9]. The presence of many other organisms is possible and depends on regional differences, the drugs injected, and laboratory analysis [11]. Microorganisms tend to be flora from the skin and oropharynx because of how the drugs are prepared and injected.

Abscesses are treated with incision and drainage under local or regional anesthesia. Drainage of an abscess may result in a large, deep wound that will heal by secondary intention. Antibiotics are prescribed pre- and postoperatively [9]. Systemic antibiotics directed against *S. aureus* and *Streptococcus* spp are generally used, including penicillinase-resistant penicillin, first-generation cephalosporins, or vancomycin [11]. Regional differences in microbial agents may also affect the antibiotic selected. Antibiotics are generally prescribed for 7 to 14 days, but the length of use can vary depending on the complexity of the case, organisms, site, and degree of concomitant cellulitis [11]. In addition to antibiotics, abscess management should include rest, elevation of the affected area, wound care, and adequate nutrition.

Chronic venous insufficiency

In the general population, common risk factors for chronic venous insufficiency (CVI) include aging (in the sixth and seventh decades of life), obesity, history of prolonged standing, deep vein thrombosis, major surgeries, immobilization, family history, pregnancy, and malignancy, to name a few factors [15–18]. Chronic venous insufficiency is estimated to affect 0.1% to 0.2% of people in developed countries, yet it is not known if injection drug users are part of these statistics [19]. In comparison with the general population, CVI develops in injection drug users in the third or fourth decade of life and affects a large number of persons [20,21]. One study [20] found a point prevalence of CVI of 87%, with 52% of those in the most advanced stages. Injection drug users risk additional complications such as repeated vein trauma, thrombophlebitis, collapsed veins, leg trauma, deep vein thrombosis, and blockage of the lymphatic system. CVI is affected by three critical factors in the legs: the condition of the veins, the ankle joint as part of the calf muscle pump, and the microcirculation.

Drug injectors may use the veins of the groin and legs because the veins of the upper body have collapsed or because injections are better able to be concealed in the lower extremities. Vascular complications to the lower extremities, including deep vein thrombosis and infections, frequently occur [22–25]. The association of injection drugs with deep vein thrombosis is as high as 21.4% for all cases of deep vein thrombosis; and this percentage increased to 52.4% for women younger than 40 years of age [26]. Deep vein thrombosis may present as clots extending centrally within the vein lumen, causing complete or partial vein blockage [22,25]. These clots may be especially marked when the groin, legs, and feet are used for injection sites. In a stuporous drug state, the muscles of the lower extremities are inactive, and a stasis of blood occurs. Nerve and muscle damage from injecting drugs may impair function of the calf muscle and ankle joint. Serious leg injury increases the risk of CVI by 2.4-fold [19]. To control pain in their legs and feet, drug injectors may not move their feet or ankle joints while walking, thus negatively affecting the calf pumping mechanism. In addition, injection drug users may experience risk factors for CVI that are similar to noninjection drug users such as surgery, heart disease, cancer, obesity, and pregnancy. Even with the presence of numerous risk factors for venous damage, research about these changes is lacking in the literature.

The treatment of CVI is the same, regardless of underlying causes, but is most critical to recognize in those who have injected in the veins of the groin, legs, and feet. Early stages of edema and skin changes can be helped with leg elevation and support stockings. When venous ulcers are present, wound care with compression dressings should be used. The person should be encouraged to walk with the normal bending motion of the ankle joint. Those who drag their feet or walk on their toes or the sides of their feet are at risk for marked deformities of foot and ankle joint, which negatively affects the calf muscle pump. Because they distrust health care, lack health insurance and access to care, and believe the wounds will eventually close, injection drug users often delay venous ulcer treatment, resulting in large wounds when the person does seek health care [21].

Issues related to wound care

There are many issues related to providing wound care to persons who have used injected drugs. This section reviews information obtained from histories of general health, social and mental health, drug use, wound assessment, and pain, and the impact that information has on wound care.

Physical health history

A review of the person's physical and mental health histories will help to determine the type of wound and its treatment and healing potential, to interpret diagnostic studies, and to identify implications of prescription medications. These persons frequently have multiple chronic health problems related to drug use such as HIV, hepatitis C, heart and liver disease, cognitive impairments, and poor nutrition [27–29], and conditions not related to drug use such as diabetes mellitus and hypertension. Nurses and other health care professionals must be careful not to stereotype a wound as drug-related without considering all possible causes. The surgical history may indicate additional risk factors for CVI. The amputation of fingers or an arm resulting from complications of drug use may affect the person's ability to participate in changing a dressing.

Psychosocial health history

The social history will provide information about where the person is living. Homeless individuals have a high rate of drug dependency [30]. If a person is living on the street or in a shelter, he or she may have difficulty carrying dressing supplies. Because the shelter may require residents to leave in the morning and not return until evening, a place to change the dressing may be lacking. Wound odor is a major concern for persons living in shelters or with family or friends. The impact of the wound in relation to the living environment must be addressed. Wound care often necessitates ongoing clinic visits. Lack of transportation is a frequent reason given for missing wound care visits [31]. Information about transportation services or reduced fare bus passes may facilitate these visits [31]. It is also important to learn about the patient's daily schedule. The person may be enrolled in drug treatment programs with required counseling sessions, have court dates, be employed, and have other home responsibilities. Depression and anxiety are commonly reported disorders among substance abusers [4]. Mental health problems can affect psychosocial functioning and may affect the person's ability to follow long-term treatment plans for wound care. Because wound care is lengthy and costly, the type of health insurance must be examined. A person who lacks health insurance should be encouraged to work with social services to apply for coverage. A descriptive note about the person's wound care can be a critical factor in obtaining health insurance. Key points of physical and psychosocial assessment are presented in Box 1.

Nutrition

Nutrition may be inadequate in persons who use drugs because of the lack of food or a place to prepare food, or because they are too high on drugs to eat. A body mass index should be calculated from the person's weight and height. A general nutrition assessment can be obtained by asking the person what typically is eaten during a day in terms of the types and amounts of food and frequency of eating. A diet high in "junk" food may provide calories but not sufficient protein or vitamins. Physiologic information can be obtained from laboratory studies such as complete blood cell count and serum albumin. Dental problems are common and can affect what a person can eat [4]. At times, the person may need vitamin and

---

Box 1. Implications of physical and psychosocial assessment

Persons who have used illicit injected drugs are at risk for
many health problems.

Health assessment should include conditions related to drug
use as well as those affecting the general population.

Health care may be affected by the person's lack of or
inadequate health insurance.

Seeking health care may be difficult for the person because of
poor mental health, chaotic life style, homelessness, lack of
transportation, fear of being stereotyped, literacy, and other
reasons.

---

iron supplements. A list of soup kitchens and their meal times is helpful to persons trying to find a place to eat. Managing nutritional deficiencies can make the difference between a wound that will or will not heal [32,33].

Drug use history

The drug use history will provide information about the use of alcohol, cigarettes, and illicit drugs. Alcohol should be examined in terms of the amount and frequency of use. Because some persons do not consider beer and wine to be alcohol, it is best to ask about beer, wine, whiskey, and spirit consumption. The National Institute on Alcohol Abuse and Alcoholism's recommendations [34] for helping patients with alcohol problems are useful for alcohol assessment and for care planning (Box 2). Because of the negative affect of alcohol on multiple body organs, it may adversely affect wound healing. Tobacco use is discussed in terms of the amount of use per day and years of use. Many economically poor individuals will minimize the impact of their smoking because of non-daily or low levels of tobacco use. Because of its negative effects on the arterial system, any cigarette use is an important assessment for arterial disease of the lower extremities. Cigarette use may negatively affect wound healing [35]. Illicit drug use is considered in terms of the drugs used and frequency and method of use. Drug addiction is a chronic illness for which a person may start and stop therapy throughout life. Injection drug use, especially when it has been injected in the groin, legs, and feet, is associated with chronic venous insufficiency at a young age [20]. Because cocaine is a vasoconstrictor, it can decrease blood supply to a wound that is trying to heal. In addition to the implications for wound care, the drug use history provides important information to consider for withdrawal manifestations if the person is hospitalized. Persons who continue to use illicit drugs should be encouraged to seek drug treatment. Information about how to enter drug treatment and support group meetings is helpful to the patient. If the person is in a methadone treatment program,

---

Box 2. Helping Patients with Alcohol Problems

To lessen risk factors for those who drink, daily limit:
   Men, no more than two drinks per day
   Women, no more than 1 drink per day
   Over 65 years of age, frail, taking medications that interact
      with alcohol, lesser amounts
A standard drink is 14 g of pure alcohol which is equal to:
   12-ounce bottle of beer or wine cooler
   5-ounce glass of wine
   1.5 ounces of spirits

   The following patients should abstain from alcohol: when
pregnant or considering pregnancy; when taking a medication
that interacts with alcohol, if alcohol dependent, if
a contraindicated medical condition or medication is present,
has reported blackouts or repeated attempts to cut down.

From National Institute on Alcohol Abuse and Alcoholism. Helping patients
with alcohol problems: a health practitioner's guide. Bethesda (MD): National
Institute on Alcohol Abuse and Alcoholism; 2004; with permission.

---

the nurse or another care provider must contact the methadone treatment center to verify the person's therapy and methadone dosage to continue methadone dosing during hospitalization.

Pain

Pain frequently occurs with infections and wounds; it is one of the most common reasons that injection drug users seek health care [36]. The treatment of pain can be extremely frustrating; health care workers have many misconceptions and value judgments about injection drug users and pain. Persons who have chronically used opioids have a decreased tolerance for pain [36]. A person's emotional response also can intensify the pain that is experienced. It is important to determine if the pain is acute and related to the abscess or wound or is chronic and related to a chronic wound or some other medical condition. Often, pain must be treated with a combination of nonsteroidal anti-inflammatory drugs and an opioid.

As with many health conditions, pain associated with CVI was ignored for many years. Pain is now recognized as occurring with CVI and is described as a dull ache or nonspecific heaviness that may be relieved with leg elevation. Pain can be present before leg ulcers develop. Because venous disease is most intense around the ankle in the lower part of the leg, the person may restrict ankle movement to decrease pain. Decreased ankle motion will negatively affect the calf muscle pump. Pain has been rated as the worst component of a leg ulcer and as severe as the pain experienced with arterial disease [37–49]. Leg ulcer pain has been identified as overwhelming, burning, shooting, and continuous. Activities such as standing and walking aggravate the pain, and sleep is impaired. Pain and mobility improve when the leg ulcer heals [38,39]. Box 3 summarizes information about pain and wounds.

Wound assessment

Substance abuse should not change the need for careful wound assessment. The wound should be assessed in terms of location, size, depth, color, drainage, odor, pain, infection, causative factors, and how the person cares for it. The wound assessment will allow the nurse and other care providers to determine the type of wound and treatment strategies. Possibly, the wound is unrelated to drug use such as a diabetic neuropathic foot ulcer or a dermatologic lesion. The presence of a wound does not necessarily mean that the person is still using illicit drugs; for example, venous ulcers may develop years after drug use has ceased.

When assessing and treating an abscess or soft tissue infection, the substances that have been injected may cause deep tissue damage that evolves over time. Initially, the wound may appear superficial but later

---

Box 3. Pain and wounds

Persons with a history of substance abuse should have pain assessed and treated.

Persons who have chronically used opioids have a decreased tolerance for pain [36].

Methadone or other maintenance therapy does not negate the need of analgesics for pain.

Treatment of wound pain is often accomplished with oral administration of a nonsteroidal anti-inflammatory drug and/or opiate such as codeine or hydrocodone with acetaminophen. Parenteral pain therapy may be needed in acute care settings. Persons with chronic wound pain may need to be referred to a pain management clinic.

In outpatient clinics, guidelines should be established for prescribing controlled substances.

The patient must be taught the proper use of analgesics as well as important side effects.

Health problems, such as liver disease, gastrointestinal bleeding, renal failure, and heavy alcohol consumption, will affect the analgesic agent that is selected.

demonstrate deeper tissue damage. The abscess may be the result of a foreign body such as a needle that broke during injecting. When an abscess is found, it must be decided if the drainage procedure can be performed in an outpatient clinic, the emergency room, or an operating room. Antibiotic therapy is an important part of abscess treatment.

Wounds are treated according to type, size, depth, and drainage. If there is depth, the wound needs to be packed. The type of packing material is dependent on the wound and what is available to the person. Gauze is probably the dressing most commonly used in the community and is moistened with normal saline and antibiotic solution or ointment or gel [50]. The wound needs to be kept moist, but moisture should not be excessive to prevent maceration of the surrounding skin.

For wounds on a lower extremity, CVI should be considered in the treatment. The edema and venous damage involved with CVI will delay the healing of surgical incisions, abscess sites, and venous ulcers. When a person presents with a wound on a lower extremity, both legs need to be examined. A person may show only the leg with the worst ulcers or the most recent wound; yet clinically, it makes sense to treat all wound problems. The nurse and other providers may feel overwhelmed because leg ulcers may be massive and multiple. Evidenced-based practice supports the use of compression therapy for the treatment of venous ulcers [32,33,51]. All brands of compression therapy are effective and should provide pressure of 30 to 40 mm Hg at the ankle. A critical issue is compliance with the dressing. The compression dressing should not be removed, rearranged, or altered, unless there is cause for concern. Wounds that are large or have odorous drainage will need the compression dressing changed at least twice per week. Ankle exercises to improve ankle joint flexion and extension may aid the calf muscle pumping action [32,33]. Routine administration of systemic antibiotics has not been found to aid ulcer healing [52], but antibiotics are used to treat infection [32,33]. The person should be encouraged to elevate the legs when sitting. Difficult situations arise in terms of edema when the person resides in a shelter where he or she must sleep in a chair. Once the ulcer has healed, the person will need to be fitted for a support stocking. The standard graduated pressure for CVI is 30 to 40 mm Hg from knee to toe. These stocking tend to be expensive and thus are not provided by some insurance plans. Because the treatment scar is weak, without a compression stocking the edema will return and the wounds may reopen. Box 4 summarizes implications for wound care.

Patient teaching

The patient should learn about the type of wound and its care. The person's readiness to learn, literacy level, and learning style are important to consider when doing patient teaching. The nurse should understand the patient's beliefs about wound care. Patients have been known to perform

> ## Box 4. Implications for wound care
>
> Wounds should be assessed in terms of type, location, size, depth, drainage, odor and infection.
>
> Wound care protocols in the community need to fit the wound type, availability of funding for supplies, the person's ability to perform care, and the living environment.
>
> Physical and psychosocial factors that may affect wound healing should be identified.
>
> Dressing selection should be based on principles of moist wound healing, wound packing for wound depth, and absorption of drainage to prevent surrounding tissue maceration from moisture.
>
> Abscess sites will need to be drained, dressing selected, and antibiotic therapy initiated.
>
> Abscesses may cause damage to surrounding tissue or organs.
>
> Soft tissue infections such as cellulitis are treated with antibiotics, generally for 7 to 14 days.
>
> Not all wounds will be related to the person's drug use, and some wounds, such as venous ulcers, may occur years after drug use has stopped.
>
> Wounds that do not heal may need to be referred for biopsy or skin graft.
>
> In working with persons with venous disease, one must assess also for the presence of arterial disease of the lower leg.

care that is negative for wound healing, such as using full-strength bleach or alcohol for wound irrigation and newspapers and magazines for dressings. For wounds from abscess sites, the person generally needs to know principles for caring for a cavity wound and monitoring for extension of the infection. For CVI, the persons should understand its chronic nature, continued vein changes with aging, and the roles of compression therapy and leg elevation. Persons who continue to inject should be encouraged not to inject in the groin or legs. Antibiotics and analgesics are frequently prescribed medications for persons with wounds. Both categories of drugs require patient teaching and are subject to diversion on the street. Antibiotic use increases concern about antimicrobial-resistant organisms. The person needs to understand the purpose of the antibiotic and the most effective way to take it. Antibiotics are used for a designated period, not the entire time of the wound. Unfortunately, the misconception of continuous antibiotic use is common street knowledge and may be reinforced by care providers who are unfamiliar with current information about chronic wound healing. Likewise with analgesics, patients need to know the proper way to take these drugs

---

Box 5. Teaching and wound care

The person should understand the cause of the wound and
    treatment methods as well as the impact of overall health
    and nutritional status on healing.
Some wounds, such as venous ulcers, may be chronic, as
    evidenced by a high risk of recurrence after healing.
Time should be provided for the person to ask questions.
Literacy will affect teaching and learning. Teaching and
    learning preferences (reading, hearing, or seeing) need to be
    determined for each person.
Reading ability, on average, is three to five grade levels below
    the number of grades of school completed [53]. Readability
    of patient teaching materials must be considered.
Persons with low literacy often feel ashamed and delay
    treatment [53].

---

and the side effects resulting from misuse. Because nonsteroidal anti-inflammatory drugs can be purchased over the counter, the patient must understand the serious side effects from these medications, especially the risks of gastrointestinal bleeding and renal failure. Box 5 summarizes teaching considerations.

Prevention

Ultimately, treating drug abuse and addiction will have the greatest impact on reducing the prevalence of wounds among current injection drug users. Full remission of drug use not withstanding, several methods can result in the occurrence of fewer wounds and perhaps less severity of the wounds that do occur. Epidemiologic studies [8,54] suggest that skin cleaning before injection reduces the likelihood of soft tissue infections. In European studies [55] of medically controlled heroin substitution, there are demonstrated skin

---

Box 6. Methods for preventing wounds among injection drug users

Provide access to clean injection equipment such as needle,
    syringe, and equipment exchange/distribution programs
Avoid sharing injection equipment
Clean the skin before injecting
Keep equipment cleaning solutions (bleach) available
Obtain access to noncontaminated drugs

---

benefits to using pharmaceutically prepared heroin. Box 6 summarizes methods to prevent wounds among injection drug users.

Summary

Persons who have injected drugs present challenges to providing wound care. They tend to have multiple physical and psychosocial problems and abuse many substances. They may mistrust health care providers because of past experiences and their perceived negative attitude toward providers. Because they often self-treat abscesses and wounds before seeking care, the infection or wound can be large. A complete history and physical examination should be obtained. All aspects of the person's background will have an impact on wound healing. Wounds need careful assessment and diagnosis. Correct diagnosis of the wound is critical for the proper treatment. Treatment decisions must also include pain control, financial concerns, living arrangements, insurance, and the person's ability to perform the care. Patient education is a critical link in enhancing positive wound healing outcomes.

References

[1] Mokdad AH, Marks JS, Stroup D, et al. Actual causes of death in the United States, 2000. JAMA 2004;291:1238–45.

[2] Schoener EP, Hopper JA, Pierre JD. Injection drug use in North America. Infect Dis Clin North Am 2002;16(2002):535–51.

[3] Summary of findings from the 1999 national household survey on drug abuse. Rockville (MD): Substance Abuse and Mental Health Services Administration; 2000.

[4] Gossop M, Marsden J, Stewart D, et al. Substance use, health and social problems of service users at 54 drug treatment agencies. Br J Psychiatry 1998;173:166–71.

[5] National Institute on Drug Abuse. Research report series heroin: abuse and addiction. Washington, D.C.: NIDA. 1997.

[6] Pieper B. Physical effects of heroin and cocaine: considerations for a wound care service. J Wound Ostomy Continence Nurs 1996;23:248–56.

[7] Binswanger IA, Kral AH, Bluthenthal RN, et al. High prevalence of abscesses and cellulitis among community-recruited injection drug users in San Francisco. Clin Infect Dis 2000;30: 579–81.

[8] Murphy EL, Devita D, Liu H, et al. Risk factors for skin and soft-tissue abscesses among injection drug users: a case-control study. Clin Infect Dis 2001;33:35–40.

[9] Bergstein JM, Baker EJ IV, Aprahamian C, et al. Soft tissue abscesses associated with parenteral drug abuse: presentation, microbiology, and treatment. Am Surg 1995;61:1105–8.

[10] Centers for Disease Control and Prevention. Soft tissue infections among injection drug users-San Francisco, California, 1996–2000. MMWR Morb Mortal Wkly Rep 2001;50(19): 381–4.

[11] Ebright JR, Pieper B. Skin and soft tissue infections in injection drug users. Infect Dis Clin North Am 2002;16:697–712.

[12] Graham CA, McNaughton GW, Crawford R. "Popping": a cause of soft tissue sepsis in chronic drug abusers. Eur J Emerg Med 1999;6(3):259–61.

[13] Henriksen BM, Albrektsen SB, Simper LB, et al. Soft tissue infections from drug abuse, a clinical and microbiological review of 145 cases. Acta Orthop Scand 1994;65:625–8.

[14] Wallace JR, Lucas CE, Ledgerwood A. Social, economic, and surgical anatomy of a drug-related abscess. Am Surg 1986;52:398–401.

[15] Geerts WH, Code KI, Jay RM, et al. A prospective study of venous thromboembolism after minor trauma. N Engl J Med 1994;331:1601–6.

[16] Graham ID, Harrison MB, Nelson A, et al. Prevalence of lower-limb ulceration: a systematic review of prevalence studies. Adv Skin Wound Care 2003;16:305–16.

[17] Weimann EE, Salzman EW. Deep vein thrombosis. N Engl J Med 1994;331:1630–41.

[18] Porter JM, Moneta GL. International consensus committee on chronic venous disease. Reporting standards in venous disease: an update. In: Glovicki P, Yao JT, editors. Handbook of venous disease. London: Chapman & Hall; 1996. p. 629–51.

[19] Scott TE, LaMort WW, Gorin DR, et al. Risk factors for chronic venous insufficiency: a dual case-control study. J Vasc Surg 1995;22:622–8.

[20] Pieper B, Templin T. Chronic venous insufficiency in persons with a history of injection drug use. Res Nurs Health 2001;24:423–32.

[21] Pieper B. A retrospective analysis of venous ulcer healing in current and former users of injected drugs. J Wound Ostomy Continence Nurs 1996;23:291–6.

[22] Kirchenbaum SE, Midenberg ML. Pedal and lower extremity complications of substance abuse. J Am Podiatry Assoc 1982;72:380–7.

[23] Mackenzie AR, Laing RB, Douglas JG, et al. High prevalence of iliofemoral venous thrombosis with severe groin infection among injecting drug users in north east Scotland: successful use of low molecular weight heparin with antibiotics. Postgrad Med J 2000; 76(899):561–5.

[24] Pardes JB, Falanga V, Kerdel FA. Delayed cutaneous ulcerations arising at sites of prior parenteral drug abuse. J Am Acad Dermatol 1993;29:1052–4.

[25] Yeager RA, Hobson RW II, Padberg FT, et al. Vascular complications related to drug abuse. J Trauma 1987;27(3):305–8.

[26] McColl MD, Tait RC, Greer IA, et al. Injecting drug use is a risk factor for deep vein thrombosis in women in Glasgow. Br J Haematol 2001;112(3):641–3.

[27] O'Connor PG, Selwyn PA, Schottenfeld RS. Medical care for injection drug users with human immunodeficiency virus infection. N Engl J Med 1994;331(7):450–9.

[28] Stein MD. Medical consequences of substance abuse. Psychiatr Clin North Am 1999;22(2): 351–70.

[29] Cherubin CE, Sapira JD. The medical complications of drug addiction and the medical assessment of the intravenous drug user: 25 years later. Ann Intern Med 1993;119:1017–28.

[30] Finnie A, Nicolson P. Injecting drug use: implications for skin and wound management. Br J Nurs 2002;11(6):s17–28.

[31] Pieper B, DiNardo E. Reasons for nonattendance for the treatment of venous ulcers in an inner-city clinic. J Wound Ostomy Continence Nurs 1998;25:180–6.

[32] Kunimoto B, Colling M, Gulliver W, et al. Best practices for the prevention and treatment of venous leg ulcers. Ostomy Wound Manage 2001;47(2):34–50.

[33] Kunimoto BT. Management and prevention of venous leg ulcers: a literature-guided approach. Ostomy Wound Manage 2001;47(6):36–49.

[34] National Institute on Alcohol Abuse and Alcoholism. Helping patients with alcohol problems: a health practitioner's guide. Bethesda (MD): National Institute on Alcohol Abuse and Alcoholism; 2004. Available at: http://www.niaaa.nih.gov/publications/Practitioner/ HelpingPatients.htm. Accessed October 21, 2004.

[35] Silverstein P. Smoking and wound healing. Am J Med 1992;93(Suppl 1A):S225–45.

[36] Hopper JA, Shafi T. Management of the hospitalized injection drug user. Infect Dis Clin North Am 2002;16(2002):571–87.

[37] Flett R, Harcourt B, Alpass F. Psychosocial aspects of chronic lower leg ulcerations in the elderly. West J Nurs Res 1994;16:183–92.

[38] Franks PJ, Bosanquet N, Brown D, et al. Perceived health in a randomized trial of treatment for chronic venous ulceration. Eur J Vasc Endovasc Surg 1999;17:155–9.

[39] Franks PJ, Moffatt CJ. Health related quality of life in patients with venous ulceration: use of the Nottingham health profile. Qual Life Res 2001;10:693–700.

[40] Hamer C, Cullum NA, Roe BH. Patients' perceptions of chronic leg ulcers. J Wound Care 1994;3:99–101.

[41] Hofman D, Ryan T, Arnold F. Pain in venous ulcers. J Wound Care 1997;6:222–4.

[42] Hyland ME, Ley A, Thomson B. Quality of life of leg ulcer patients: questionnaire and preliminary findings. J Wound Care 1994;3:294–8.

[43] Krasner D. Painful venous ulcers: themes and stories about living with the pain and suffering. J Wound Ostomy Continence Nurs 1998;25:158–68.

[44] Phillips T, Stanton B, Provan A, et al. A study of the impact of leg ulcers on quality of life: financial, social, and psychologic implications. J Am Acad Dermatol 1994;31:49–53.

[45] Price P, Harding K. Measuring health-related quality of life in patients with chronic leg ulcers. Wounds 1996;8:91–4.

[46] Walshe C. Living with a venous leg ulcer: a descriptive study of patients' experiences. J Adv Nurs 1995;22:1092–100.

[47] Walters SJ, Morrell CJ, Dixon S. Measuring health-related quality of life in patients with venous leg ulcers. Qual Life Res 1999;8:327–36.

[48] Pieper B, Rossi R, Templin T. Pain associated with venous ulcers in injecting drug use. Ostomy Wound Manage 1998;44(11):54–67.

[49] Pieper B, Szczepaniak K, Templin T. Psychosocial adjustment, coping, and quality of life in persons with venous ulcers and a history of intravenous drug use. J Wound Ostomy Continence Nurs 2000;27:227–39.

[50] Pieper B, Templin TN, Dobal M, et al. Wound prevalence, types, and treatment in home care. Adv Wound Care 1999;12:117–26.

[51] Nelson EA, Cullum N, Jones J. Venous leg ulcers. In: Godlee F, executive editor. Clinical evidence concise. London: BMJ Pubishing Group; 2003. p. 410–1.

[52] Alinovi A, Bassissi P, Pini M. Systemic administration of antibiotics in the management of venous ulcers. A randomized clinical trial. J Am Acad Dermatol 1986;15:186–91.

[53] Lee PP. Why literacy matters. Arch Ophthalmol 1999;117:100–3.

[54] Vlahov D, Sullivan M, Astemborski J, et al. Bacterial infections and skin cleaning prior to injection among intravenous drug users. Public Health Rep 1992;107(5):595–8.

[55] Conrad CT, Steffen T. Development of skin diseases in intravenous drug dependent patients treated with heroin substitution. Schweiz Rundsch Med Prax 2000;89:1899–906.

ELSEVIER
SAUNDERS

Nurs Clin N Am 40 (2005) 365–389

NURSING
CLINICS
OF NORTH AMERICA

Pressure Ulcers: The Great Insult

JoAnn Maklebust, MSN, APRN-BC, AOCN, FAAN

*Department of Oncologic Surgery, Karmanos Cancer Institute, Detroit Medical Center,
4100 John R, Detroit, MI 48201, USA*

Pressure ulcers are a clinically significant and costly health care problem. A pressure ulcer, sometimes called a decubitus ulcer or bedsore, is defined as any lesion caused by unrelieved pressure that damages underlying tissue. Pressure ulcers are found most frequently in soft tissue over bony prominences exposed to compressing surfaces [1]. More than 95% of all pressure ulcers occur on the lower half of the body. The greatest number of ulcers occurs within the pelvic girdle because it is the heaviest part of the human body. Areas prone to pressure ulcers include the sacrum, greater trochanter of the femur, ischial tuberosity, lateral malleolus, calcaneus, occiput, chin, elbow, scapula, and iliac crest [2–4]. Pressure ulcers can range in severity from blanchable erythema of intact skin to deep tissue damage involving muscle and bone. Because pressure is the primary cause of skin injury over bony prominences, the term pressure ulcer is preferred to such synonyms as bedsore or decubitus ulcer [4,5]. Because the origin and treatment differ, it is important to distinguish among pressure ulcers resulting from other conditions, such as venous ulcers, arterial ulcers, and diabetic foot ulcers.

This article provides an updated summary of the current pressure ulcer literature. Rather than providing new material, many recent articles review information found in the Agency for Healthcare Research and Quality (AHRQ) (formerly known as the Agency for Health Care Policy and Research) Clinical Practice Guidelines on Pressure Ulcer Prevention and Treatment [6,7]. These articles discuss pressure ulcer causes, staging, risk factors, risk assessment tools, pressure ulcer prevention and treatment, and ulcer-related pain [8–10]. A review of these articles will not be repeated here because many of them are updated and well covered elsewhere in this issue on wound care. This article focuses on recent pressure ulcer literature that is more controversial in nature. Current literature particularly emphasizes

E-mail address: JMacklebu@dmc.org

revisiting the causes and natural history of pressure ulcers [11,12], pressure ulcer staging systems [13–16], whether pressure ulcers are preventable [17–20], and whether all of them will heal [20–25].

Also of note is the increased interest in pressure ulcers by governmental agencies and regulating bodies [26–28]. There are many recent articles on quality of care related to patient safety, quality improvement strategies for pressure ulcer management, pressure ulcer surveillance methods, and regulatory oversight [29–31].

Pressure ulcer causes

Unrelieved pressure is the most important factor in the pathogenesis of pressure ulcers [2–4]. Pressure ulceration is the clinical manifestation of cellular necrosis caused by vascular insufficiency in an area under pressure. When transient pressure interrupts blood flow, the skin becomes pale. If the ischemia lasts for more than 1 minute, the localized area becomes red or hyperemic, and blanchable erythema occurs; this is believed to be a reversible phenomenon. Nonblanchable erythema suggests capillary extravasation of plasma and red cells into the tissue, and it may be reversible if it is promptly recognized. Subcutaneous tissues, including muscles, are more sensitive to ischemia than the epidermis and dermis [32]. Hence, pressure ulcers are more extensive than they appear superficially. One of the difficulties in studying pressure ulcer causation is that seldom does an individual receive a clinically significant pressure insult when he or she is not at high risk for both the development of a pressure ulcer and additional pressure insults. This makes it difficult to separate one exposure from all other exposures that may contribute to pressure ulceration. Versluysen [33], who studied elderly patients with hip fractures, attempted to determine the length of time between the pressure insult and pressure ulceration. The pressure insult was believed to have occurred during operative repair of the hip fracture. The study found that the greatest incidence of new onset postoperative pressure ulcers occurred within the first 2 postoperative days, although, some new onset pressure damage was noted as many as 5 to 7 days postoperatively. These results and the results of others [34,35] suggest that pressure wounds occur within the first 2 days after the insult and that wounds occurring beyond this time frame are caused by continuous soft tissue insults in high risk populations. A clinically significant pressure insult may go undetected for as many as 7 days. A study by Allman et al [36] followed a cohort of immobile, hospitalized patients for several weeks to assess the development of pressure ulcers. Most pressure ulcers were noted within the first 2 weeks of hospitalization. Stage I pressure ulcers were found to be an independent risk factor for the development of Stages II and III pressure ulcers. Although no direct attempt was made to identify an isolated incident of clinically significant pressure insult, this study did show that the rate of development of new pressure ulcers appeared to peak during the second week of hospitalization. These data may imply that isolated, clinically significant episodes of pressure insults are uncommon and that pressure ulcer causation is dependent on multiple insults to a high risk host. Readers are referred to a previous issue of *Nursing Clinics of North America* [5] and several recent textbooks [32,37–41] for a more comprehensive review of pressure ulcer causes.

Epidemiology

The available data regarding prevalence, incidence, and impact of pressure ulcers suggest that they are a serious public health problem in the United States. These ulcers can lead to devastating complications and place demands on an already stressed health care system. Pressure ulcers promise to become an even bigger issue as the U.S. population ages. Pressure ulcers are common among the elderly, in the community, and in acute and long-term care settings. Confinement to a bed or chair for a week has been found to increase the prevalence of pressure ulceration by 28%. When a Stage I pressure ulcer develops, the risk for additional ulcers on the same individual is reported to increase ten-fold [4].

The exact prevalence of patients with pressure ulcers is not known. Estimates of pressure ulcer incidence and prevalence vary widely because of different methods of data collection, patient care settings, and types of subjects. The National Pressure Ulcer Advisory Panel (NPUAP, available at: http://www.NPUAP.org) published [42] the most comprehensive review of pressure ulcer incidence and prevalence studies in 2001. Large multisite studies performed across the United States over the last 10 years reported a pressure ulcer prevalence ranging from 10% to18% in acute care, 2.3% to 28% in long-term care facilities, and 0% to 29% in the community. Pressure ulcer incidence rates also have wide variation. Pressure ulcer incidence ranges from 0.4% to 38% in acute care, 2.2% to 23.9% in long-term care, and 0% to 17% in home care. Valid comparisons cannot be made among these studies or to data before 1990 because of methodological differences. These figures should not be considered as benchmarks to determine acceptable pressure ulcers rates for a given setting [41].

The prevalence of pressure ulcers among certain populations such as ICU patients or spinal cord injured and rehabilitation center patients is particularly high. Younger adults with spinal injuries are especially vulnerable [43]. There also is some evidence that different skin pigmentations may be more sensitive to pressure than others. Meehan [44] reported a disproportionate (16%) number of severe Stage IV ulcers in black patients in hospitals. Ayello and Lyder [45] reported that people with darkly pigmented skin had the lowest prevalence of Stage I pressure ulcers but the highest prevalence of Stage II to IV ulcers. It is not known whether this is caused by tissue sensitivity or because the ulcers were not as easily recognized in early development.

Pressure ulcer classification systems

The literature discusses many classification systems for grading or staging pressure ulcers. Most are based on the system developed in 1975 by Shea [46], who believed that a pathology-based pressure ulcer classification system would simplify communication for all health care disciplines. This staging system primarily describes ulcer depth. In earlier work, Shea also included a "closed pressure ulcer" in the schema. Over the years, Shea's original work was modified: in 1989, the NPUAP held a pressure ulcer consensus development conference at which attendees reached consensus on a revised pressure ulcer classification system [13]. Over time, it was determined by clinicians that in addition to depth, color definitions in the staging systems were not appropriate for all skin tones [47]. An NPUAP task force [48] was formed to continue refining the pressure ulcer staging system to clarify Stage I ulcers in persons with darkly pigmented skin. It is the most commonly used system in use today.

- Stage I is characterized by an observable pressure-related alteration of intact skin which, when compared with an adjacent or opposite site area on the body, may include changes in one or more of the following: skin temperature (warmth or coolness); tissue consistency (firm or boggy feel); or sensation (pain, itching). The ulcer appears as a defined area of persistent redness in lightly pigmented skin; in darker skin tones the ulcer may appear with persistent red, blue, or purple hues.
- Stage II is characterized by a partial thickness skin loss involving the epidermis or dermis. The ulcer is superficial and presents clinically as an abrasion, blister, or shallow crater.
- Stage III is characterized by a full thickness skin loss involving damage or necrosis of subcutaneous tissue that may extend down to, but not through the underlying fascia. The ulcer presents clinically as a deep crater with or without undermining of the adjacent tissue.
- Stage IV is characterized by a full thickness skin loss with extensive destruction, tissue necrosis, or damage to the muscle, bone, or supporting structures.

Pressure ulcers covered by eschar and slough cannot be staged until the necrotic tissue is removed and the ulcer base can be seen [7,8]. Pressure ulcers also can be characterized on the basis of features other than depth, for example, on size, color, or the presence of necrotic tissue, and undermining of tissue. There is discussion by the NPUAP about revisiting the current pressure ulcer staging system to further clarify definitions [11].

Darkly pigmented skin

Most pressure ulcer staging system definitions emphasize intact skin redness to indicate pressure damage [7,8,46]. Skin color is influenced by the presence of skin pigments such as melanin or hemosiderin, making it difficult to identify pressure-related changes in patients with darkly pigmented skin [32]. Dark skin does not exhibit the characteristic erythematous changes normally associated with pressure damage in lightly pigmented skin. As a general rule, damaged areas of skin tend to look darker than surrounding skin and often are indurated, edematous, taut, and shiny. Color changes in dark skin can range from purplish to blue, comparable with a red to reddish-blue color associated with erythema in lighter skin tones. The high melanin concentration in dark skin prevents the observation of the blanch response to light finger pressure. If compressed, the color of pressure-related damage does not pale or blanch [32]. Matas et al [49] studied the ability of visible and near infrared spectroscopy to monitor a blanch response in light and dark skin, based on changes in blood volume. The light and dark-skinned groups differed in pigmentation in both visible and near infrared regions of the spectrum.

Refined clinical assessment skills are required to detect early signs of pressure-related changes in dark skin. One of the most reliable indications of ischemic damage is a localized area of damaged skin that feels warm to the touch, especially when compared with the surrounding skin. This temperature is caused by the inflammatory process and is best detected by lightly touching the affected area with the back of the hand or fingers. If pressure is unrelieved and further tissue damage is allowed to occur, the area of warmth eventually will feel cooler than surrounding skin, indicating that ischemic changes have occurred. In a repeated measures design, Sprigle et al [50] found that increased and decreased temperature differences can be used to indicate reactive hyperemia or Stage I pressure ulcers. The research team tested the skin temperature and appearance of 65 patients presenting with pressure-induced erythema over bony prominences. Warmth or coolness was present in 85% of the erythematous sites on patients with Stage I ulcers.

Skin temperature changes of erythematous areas are slight and can be better detected without the use of gloves and in natural light. Skin assessment for erythema should not be made with fluorescent lighting because it tends to impart blue tones to dark skin. To provide a more comprehensive and culturally sensitive definition of pressure damage to dark intact skin, the NPUAP task force on "Stage I Definition and Darkly Pigmented Skin" chose to include more than color [48]. Task force members revised the definition of Stage I pressure ulcers to include additional indicators of warmth, tissue consistency, or sensation.

Deep tissue injury

Current pressure ulcer staging definitions and the implications of "deep purple lesions" over bony prominences are controversial. In individuals with lighter skin, deep purple coloration is characteristic of microcirculatory changes. Parish et al [32] explain that the upper portion of dermis is sufficiently transparent for color from deeper tissues to be observed. In deep tissue, blue is more easily transmitted than red; hence, dilated blood vessels in the deep dermis often appear to be blue. Erythematous purplish lesions on patients with intact skin who ultimately develop full thickness Stage III to IV pressure ulcers are believed to be indicative of deep tissue injury. The NPUAP Deep Tissue Injury Task Force [11] identified and critically evaluated 158 relevant articles on how experts and researchers in the pressure ulcer field view deep tissue injury. The review concentrated on both recent and historical reports known to pressure ulcer experts. There are disagreements on how to assess Stage I pressure ulcers because there is no international grading system. Purple pressure-related skin changes are sometimes considered to be Stage I or superficial, and sometimes they are considered full thickness tissue damage [51]. There is contention about whether Stage I ulcers are characterized by blanching or nonblanching erythema, whether damage starts at the epidermis or deeper at the interface of soft tissue and bone, and whether these ulcers are reversible. The NPUAP publication "Pressure-related Deep Tissue Injury Under Intact Skin and the Current Pressure Ulcer Staging Systems" [11] recommends how clinicians should describe a pressure-related injury to subcutaneous tissue under intact skin (these lesions may herald the subsequent development of Stage III or IV pressure ulcers, even with optimal management) and how researchers should investigate deep tissue injury. The article reviews the way in which the commonly cited pressure ulcer staging systems and experts describe this entity and includes NPUAP commentary on the presumed pathophysiology of these lesions. Guidelines are given for delineating deep tissue injury from superficial tissue injury. NPUAP authors also include ways in which clinicians and researchers can become involved in investigations that will lead to improved understanding of the epidemiology, natural history, and treatment of these pressure injuries. The Ninth Biennial NPUAP conference (February 25–26, 2005) [11] highlighted the realities of the current pressure ulcer staging system. A consensus process was used to develop criteria for Stages I and II pressure ulcers. It was suggested that deep tissue injury be reclassified as a type of Stage I pressure ulcer. Findings from this important conference will modify our current understanding and definition of Stage I pressure ulcers. In turn, revised definitions will demand better documentation of this entity and force us to propose appropriate treatments. Work on deep tissue injury has clinical, regulatory, and legal implications for the future.

Risk assessment

Most pressure ulcers are preventable if patient risk is recognized in time for preventive actions to be initiated. Identifying persons at high risk for pressure ulcers is vital [52]. The pressure ulcer clinical practice guidelines [6–8,53] developed by the AHRQ, Wound Ostomy Continence Nurses Society, and American Medical Directors Association recommend systematic use of a risk assessment tool such as the Braden Scale for Predicting Pressure Sore Risk [54]. The Braden Scale is a formal, internationally recognized tool with high reliability in predicting patients at risk for pressure ulcers and thus provides a first step in the prevention of pressure ulcers. The Braden Scale evaluates the level of sensory perception, skin moisture, physical activity, mobility, nutrition, friction, and shear. Each of these subscales is rated from 1 to 4 except friction and shear, which are rated from 1 to 3. Each rating is accompanied by a brief description of the criteria for assigning the rating. When the six subscales are added together, the total Braden Scale score ranges from 6 to 23. A lower Braden Scale score indicates that patients are at higher risk for developing pressure ulcers. A cut-off score of 18 or below in an adult patient is considered predictive of pressure ulceration unless preventive measures are taken. The Braden Scale has been tested in a variety of settings to determine if different cut-off scores should be used with different patient populations [55–61]. Lyder [47] examined the predictive ability of the Braden Scale in a population of African American and Asian patients and found that a cut-off score of 18 provided the most accurate prediction of pressure ulcer risk. Collective evidence thus far indicates that a cut-off score of 18 should be used for clinical practice in all settings and with all ethnic groups [62,63].

Use of the Braden Scale is intended to allow nurse providers to reliably score a patient's level of risk for developing pressure ulcers. It should be used to screen patients who are bed or wheelchair bound and are therefore predisposed to pressure ulcers. Many health care facilities require that nurses use the Braden Scale to evaluate patient risk for developing pressure ulcers. Hergenroeder et al [64] placed a question on the hospital admission database asking nurses, "Is the patient at risk for pressure ulcers?" Initially, the investigators were disappointed to find that nurses often left the question blank. Researchers independently rated patient risk by using the Braden Scale and then compared their risk score with nursing judgment. A direct query to nurses demonstrated a correlation between Braden Scale and nurses judgment, but only patients who were at moderate to high risk on the Braden Scale were identified as being at risk by nursing judgment. Salvadena et al [65] found that when nurses predicted risk only as "yes" or "no," preventive actions were taken only 27% of the time.

To increase the accuracy of pressure ulcer risk assessment, the Advanced Practice Nurses (APNs) and Wound Ostomy Continence Nurses (WOCNs) at the Detroit Medical Center developed and tested a computer-based learning module to help nurses learn how to correctly use the Braden Scale [66]. Detroit Medical Center (DMC) nurses are required to enroll in yearly computer-based Braden Scale competency testing through case study exemplars for acute, long-term, and home care, the emergency department, and the operating room. Nurses must correctly calculate the total Braden Scale score and each Braden Subscale score. Knowledge of patients' Braden

Subscale scores helps nurses plan appropriate pressure ulcer prevention measures. The Braden Scale learning module tests nurses' ability to select interventions based on ameliorating risk factors identified by Braden Subscale scores. The recommendations for preventing pressure ulcers include risk assessment, measures to relieve pressure, friction and shear, adequate nutrition, proper skin care nutrition, and steps to minimize moisture from urinary and fecal incontinence [6,8,53,62,63,67].

Fisher et al [68] reported results from a study that investigated the association between Braden risk assessment subscale scores and hospitalized adults with pressure ulcers. Factors associated with pressure ulcers were advanced age, male gender, sensory perception, moisture, mobility, nutrition, and friction and shear. Three interactions also were found to be associated with pressure ulcers. Age, sensory perception, moisture, and sensory perception were negatively associated with pressure ulcers, whereas nutrition and male gender were positively associated with pressure ulcers. These findings highlight the need for early intensive preventive measures for older patients and for patients with deficits related to sensory perception, moisture, shearing forces, and nutrition (in males) [68]. This study also demonstrates the use and importance of Braden subscales scores.

Are all pressure ulcers preventable?

Pressure ulcer prevention is one of the most important clinical issues in long-term care. There is great debate among experienced clinicians about whether all pressure ulcers are preventable. In a recent editorial, Glover [17] posed the question, "Are pressure ulcers preventable?" The author noted that, "The debate is heating up." The debate centers on whether pressure ulcers result from factors largely dependent on caregivers or whether pressure ulcers result from factors associated with patient morbidity. Thomas [18], a geriatrician, discusses opposing answers to the question "Are pressure ulcers avoidable?" The discussion asserts that this debate is critical because the emphasis in reducing the incidence of pressure ulcers depends on which view predominates. Pressure ulcer prevention and quality improvement strategies are aimed at reducing pressure ulcer incidence; yet, epidemiologic data demonstrate stability in the incidence of pressure ulcers despite regulatory oversight and improvements in available pressure ulcer prevention technology. The explanation for this stable incidence includes either "a failure of known effective preventive treatment or the failure of prevention strategies to be effective in spite of being applied. No intervention has been reported that consistently and reproducibly reduces pressure ulcer incidence to zero. The published data on pressure ulcer prevention do not support an assumption that all pressure ulcers are preventable. An effective strategy demonstrated to eliminate pressure ulcers across health care settings is lacking" [18].

Agreeing with this view, Witkowski and Parish [20] assert that the pressure ulcer may not be preventable or even curable. Preventable pressure ulcers are those that occur in low-risk patients. Referring to pressure ulcers in the aged and terminally ill as "unpreventable" or "permissible" ulcers, they state that no amount of attention or skill on the part of the caregiver will avert this untoward occurrence in some high-risk patients. "Decubitus ulcers can be part of the syndrome of multiple organ failure. Some risk factors are irreversible, despite good care. If the heart, lungs or kidneys are failing, it is not logical to believe that the integument will not. Deterioration of the skin as a terminal event is understated and underestimated. There are no known medications, procedures or suitable biological or mechanical replacements to sustain or enhance cutaneous function. Keeping frail, sick people alive longer has uncovered a new set of illnesses one of which is the bedsore that is occurring with increasing frequency. Until more effective preventive measures are discovered, we must discard the fallacy that all decubitus ulcers are preventable" [20].

Carrying on this debate, Brandeis et al [19] queried pressure ulcer experts about this question. The investigators mailed 92 36-item questionnaires to experts in the field to determine their opinion regarding the preventability of pressure ulcers, the resources available for prevention in nursing homes, and the role of negligence lawsuits in pressure ulcer care. Sixty-five of the 92 surveys were completed and returned. Sixty-two percent of the respondents disagreed with the statement that all pressure ulcers were preventable. Only 5% said that nursing homes had adequate resources to prevent pressure ulcers. Most respondents disagreed that pressure ulcers were necessarily signs of neglect, and they also disagreed that nursing homes should be sued when a resident develops a pressure ulcer.

In an editorial, Olshansky [69] takes an opposing view and advocates a new approach to pressure ulcer prevention. "We have gone wrong, not through lack of knowledge, but rather, lack of implementation. The prevention process should begin with a root cause analysis to answer these questions: Why do patients develop pressure ulcers in intensive care units? Is it lack of knowledge or are there too few nurses? Are nurses too busy saving the patient's life to the extent that pressure ulcer prevention becomes secondary and patients are not turned? Are more pressure-reducing/relieving beds needed or necessary? Are the support surfaces we use effective? Is more physician participation needed in the care process? Should more accountability for quality issues be required? What are quality outcomes regarding pressure ulcer prevention? What is the incidence of pressure ulcers in our institutions over the last 10 years? Is it improving? Worsening? Staying the same? What is the quality review process when a patient develops a pressure ulcer? How many institutions use benchmarks and clinical pathways for their pressure ulcer prevention? Does staff have the core knowledge needed to achieve high quality outcomes? Hard questions, certainly, but basic to ensuring the ability to implement appropriate preventive measures. Once answers to these questions are ascertained, another question undoubtedly will follow: Why aren't doctors and nurses taking the necessary steps to prevent ulcers in our sophisticated hospitals and nursing homes when we have the knowledge to do so? In its recent report Priority Areas of National Action: Transforming Health Care Quality, the Institute of Medicine observes, 'We spend more than $1 trillion on health care annually, we have extraordinary knowledge and capacity to deliver the best care in the world, but we repeatedly fail to translate that knowledge and capacity into clinical practice. It is time to tap the resources of available experts and address the issue of preventing pressure ulcers in a positive, scientific, and caring way, and translate our knowledge of pressure ulcer prevention into practice. It is time for all of us to direct our energy and resources to solving the problem so the question, Could this ulcer have been prevented? becomes irrelevant' " [69].

Will all pressure ulcers heal?

In a retrospective analysis of pressure ulcer quality-assurance data, Brown [23] ascertained the relationship between the occurrence of nosocomial full thickness pressure ulcers, healing, and mortality. Start day was the day that the ulcer was determined to have occurred, and end day was the date the patient was pronounced dead. Major diagnoses for all patients were cerebrovascular accident, diabetes, and cancer. The majority of ulcers were located in the sacral-coccygeal area (66.2%) and heel (16.2%). None of the ulcers healed in patients who died within 180 days of ulcer onset. A 180-day mortality rate of 68.9% was noted in people who developed nosocomial full thickness pressure ulcers. Other pressure ulcer experts agree that not all pressure ulcers are curable, especially in terminally ill patients [18,20]. Many factors can negatively affect the wound-healing process, leading to recalcitrant wounds. Tissue perfusion, debridement, and wound fluid management all have an impact on healing. Biochemical and cellular commonalities can be identified across a number of wound causes. Healing data for various acute and chronic wounds, including pressure ulcers, fail to show significant differences in times to healing. The author challenged clinicians to consider the healing process at a biochemical level even when at the bedside [24].

Some authors proposed that with good medical care, pressure ulcers can be expected to heal. Prospective data from 19,889 elderly residents of 51 nursing homes were analyzed to determine the prevalence, incidence, and natural history of pressure ulcers. Among all residents admitted to nursing homes, 11.3% possessed a Stage II to IV pressure ulcer. For those residents admitted to the nursing home without pressure ulcers during the study period, the 1-year incidence was 13.2%. This increased to 21.6% by 2 years of nursing home stay. People already residing at the nursing home at the start of the study had a 1-year incidence of 9.5% that increased to 20.4% by

2 years. Longitudinal follow-up of residents with pressure ulcers demonstrated that a majority of their ulcers were healed by 1 year. Most of the improvement occurred early in a person's nursing home stay. Although nursing home residents have a higher mortality, with good medical care pressure ulcers can be expected to heal [22,29]. Are we asking the right questions when we ask if all pressure ulcer will heal? Ennis [25] posed the questions of whether we can, must, or should try to heal all wounds. Wound healing may be preferred, but it may not always be possible or appropriate. Healing may be way down on the list of things that the patient needs to improve their quality of life. The multidisciplinary team, "For the Recognition of the Adult, Immobilized Life," (FRAIL) [25] is attempting to legitimize the concept of nonhealable wounds, establish "permission" for treatment strategies with nonhealing endpoints, highlight palliative elements of nonhealing treatments, and identify gaps for products and services that support nonhealing strategies.

Healing scales

Pressure ulcer staging systems are erroneously used to monitor and describe pressure ulcer healing. This practice, known as reverse- or down-staging, is not recommended [70]. Full thickness ulcers do not heal by progressing inversely from a deep to a more shallow stage; instead, they heal through a process that includes granulation, wound contraction, re-epithelialization, and scar formation [14,70]. Because pressure ulcer staging systems were being misused by reversing the numeric order (eg, Stage IV to III to II to I) to indicate healing, several new tools have been advocated. The Pressure Sore Status Tool (PSST) [71], the Pressure Ulcer Scale for Healing (PUSH) tool [72], the Sessing Scale [73], and the Wound Healing Scale (WHS) [74] have been proposed as alternatives to the use of reverse staging. The PUSH tool [75] is pragmatic in that it contains three assessment items that when added together indicate the amount and direction of wound healing. The healing process is described by changes in surface area, extent of necrotic tissue and exudate, and the presence of granulation tissue. Training in the use of this scale is required to ensure that ulcers are assessed in a consistent manner. The PUSH tool was tested on the post-acute care minimum data set (MDS) and is now being considered by the Center for Medicare and Medicaid Services for inclusion in section M of the MDS for nursing homes [41]. The MDS is a federal document used to screen patients by all 17,000 nursing homes in the United States.

Patient safety and pressure ulcers

Patient safety is an issue of major national interest. Policymakers, providers, and consumers have made the safety of care in United States a top priority [26–28]. The need to assess, monitor, track, and improve the safety of inpatient care became apparent with the publication of the Institute of Medicine's series of reports [31] describing the problem of medical errors. As our health care system becomes more complex, the possibility of significant adverse effects increases. Pressure ulcers are one of the most frequently mentioned negative patient outcomes. Pressure ulcers also are frequently indicated on computerized hospital discharge abstracts from the AHRQ Healthcare Cost and Use Project [74]. This indicator is intended to flag cases of in-hospital pressure ulcers. Its definition is limited to pressure ulcer as a secondary diagnosis to better screen cases that may present on admission. Additionally, this indicator excludes patients who have a length of stay of 4 days or less because it is unlikely that a pressure ulcer would develop within this period of time. This indicator also excludes patients who are particularly susceptible to pressure ulcer, such as patients with major skin disorders and paralysis. Berlowitz [76], in an eloquent editorial, encourages health care professionals to "Strive for Six Sigma" in caring for pressure ulcers (Box 1).

Health care provider knowledge about pressure ulcers

Xakellis et al [83] showed that implementing guideline-based pressure ulcer prevention protocols presents a major leadership challenge. These researchers assert that translating pressure ulcer guidelines into practice is harder than it sounds. Implementing education and protocols at a long-term care facility did demonstrate an initial reduction in the incidence of pressure ulcers, but these reductions were lost over time. The authors warn that prevention protocols may be abandoned if there is not a skin care champion to reward staff for implementing pressure ulcer prevention measures. Although nursing personnel have primary responsibility for skin care and pressure ulcer prevention programs, preventing pressure ulcers also requires leadership and commitment from the nursing administration. A large tertiary care hospital reported [84] success in decreasing nosocomial pressure ulcers by using the skills and knowledge of all their nursing leaders and staff nurses. It is unclear whether the decrease in the incidence of pressure ulcers was sustained.

Pieper et al [85] determined that nurses were lacking in routine use and documentation of pressure ulcer risk assessment and pressure ulcer prevention methods. Pieper and Mott [86] further demonstrated that health care professionals' knowledge about pressure ulcers needed to be updated. The authors found that educational content about pressure ulcers needed to be integrated into nursing and medical school curricula. As of 1991, undergraduate nursing students and nursing staff had little exposure to skin integrity problems through nursing textbooks, which was recognized as a hindrance to pressure ulcer education in American nursing schools.

Nursing students were exposed to as little as 200 lines of text and very few charts or illustrations about pressure ulcers during their education. This suggested that undergraduate nurses' knowledge base about pressure ulcers was very limited [87]. A review of updated editions of these nursing textbooks reveals a wide variation in the number of lines of text devoted to pressure ulcers, the depth and quality of information, and the number of illustrations and tables. New findings include both cultural concepts and the results of research studies. A survey of the majority of current nursing textbooks shows improvement in the amount and quality of pressure ulcer information, and the investigators have suggested specific pressure ulcer content for future nursing textbooks [88].

Pressure ulcers recently were chosen as a target condition for quality improvement in geriatric care and identified as a core subject for undergraduate and graduate medical education. A small cohort of geriatric fellows was surveyed about their knowledge and confidence in caring for geriatric patients with pressure ulcers [89]. When queried, they could name some risk conditions but did not recognize the Braden Scale as a screening tool for pressure ulcer risk. The investigators concluded that the fellows needed considerable improvement in their knowledge and confidence to become clinicians and educators on the subject of pressure ulcers. To improve the quality of future geriatricians, the authors recommend specific and consistent curricular guidelines for pressure ulcer management [90].

Third- and fourth-year undergraduate students at a public university in Brazil were asked to identify extracurricular activities (eg, reading journals and articles and using the Internet to enhance comprehension of pressure ulcer care) and complete a "Pressure Ulcer Knowledge" test [91]. Students correctly answered 67.7% of the "Pressure Ulcer Knowledge" test items. Students who participated in extracurricular activities and used the Internet had significantly higher knowledge of pressure ulcer scores than those who did not. Reading did not significantly affect the knowledge test score. Generally, it was found that students had low pressure ulcer knowledge scores, but educational programs and use of the Internet were seen as having the potential to positively affect nursing students' knowledge of pressure ulcers.

Another study [92] evaluated the effects of a pressure ulcer education program for 20 Swedish nurses' knowledge of pressure ulcer risk, routine use of prevention strategies, and documentation about pressure ulcer management. Knowledge of pressure ulcer management was assessed by a questionnaire distributed to course participants immediately before and after the education program. Nursing documentation was also audited before and after education. To gain information on routine use of prevention strategies, head nurses were interviewed and the patients' care was observed before education. A nurse questionnaire was completed at an 8-month follow-up. The results showed that knowledge of pressure ulcer risk, prevention, and documentation was unsatisfactory before the education program. However,

Box 1. Strive for Six Sigma in Pressure Ulcer Care[a]

The landmark report by the Institute of Medicine, To Err is Human
[26] has focused national attention on the problem of patient
safety. The development of a pressure ulcer may represent
a common medical error. The knowledge to prevent most
pressure ulcers exists. All too often, though, this knowledge
is not translated into effective clinical practice, resulting in
significant morbidity and mortality for frail elderly patients. It
should come as no surprise that improving the prevention
and treatment of pressure ulcers in long-term care was
selected as one of the top 10 goals for national quality
improvement by the Strategic Framework Board for the
National Quality Measurement and Reporting System [28].
Chassin [77] has challenged the medical community to
commit to an industrial standard of quality improvement, the
quest for six-sigma quality [77]. Six sigma refers to the number
of standard deviations from the mean and implies that there
will be fewer than 3.4 defects per million occurrences.
How are we doing in pressure ulcer preventive care? Two reports
by Bates-Jensen et al. and other recent studies [78,79]
document that we have a long way to go. Key processes of
care, such as performing a standardized assessment to identify
at-risk patients, repositioning patients every 2 to 3 hours, and
using pressure-reducing surfaces, are often not performed.
For many of these processes, one must conclude that care is
only at the one- or two-sigma level. Errors that place nursing
home residents at significant risk occur every day. Reports by
Bates-Jensen et al. are alarming in that they suggest that many
of the currently used approaches to assessing the quality of
pressure ulcer care are inadequate. One such approach relies
on medical record reviews to determine whether important
processes of care are being performed. Bates-Jensen et al.
found little correlation between what was in the medical
record and what was directly observed [78]. The observed
use of a pressure-reducing surface often did not agree with
the medical record, and a wireless thigh monitor designed to
detect movements of the limb demonstrated long intervals
(from 4 to 11 hours) without any repositioning despite chart
documentation of a scheduled repositioning program. If these
results are generalizable to most nursing homes in this
country, it would suggest that medical-record based reviews
are not adequate for assessing the quality of pressure ulcer

care. Because of the difficulties in detecting the performance of routine processes of care in nursing homes, outcome measures have often been advocated as the preferred approach to quality measurement [80,81]. To this end, quality indicators based on pressure ulcer prevalence rates have been developed, and the Centers for Medicare and Medicaid Services routinely disseminate results on most nursing homes in this country on their Web site. Consumers throughout the country are being encouraged to use these data on pressure ulcer prevalence. The results of Bates-Jensen et al. also call into question this approach. In examining a sample of nursing homes with high and low pressure ulcer prevalence rates, they found few differences in the processes of care, not only by chart review, but also by direct observation [79]. This inability to link process and outcome measures could raise questions about the validity of the prevalence rate as a quality measure and its use as a national quality indicator. Rates of pressure ulcer development (incidence) rather than prevalence may be preferable for assessing nursing home quality [82].

Clearly, additional studies are required. Achieving six-sigma quality in pressure ulcer care will not be easy. Consider the simple task of repositioning patients every 2 hours, one of the most basic and important tasks in pressure ulcer prevention. For a nursing home with 50 at-risk patients, this implies 600 turns each day, 18,000 each month, and 216,000 each year. Six-sigma quality implies that there will be only one failure to reposition a patient each year. I doubt there is any health care facility in the country that is currently able to ensure this level of quality. It should be noted that the consistent and timely implementation of other key aspects of pressure ulcer care might currently be more feasible. How nursing homes implement best practices for pressure ulcer prevention remains uncertain. As emphasized in the Institute of Medicine report, system redesigns are usually required to ensure safe and high quality care. This is certainly the case for pressure ulcers. Although the exact design of a safe system with regard to the prevention of pressure ulcers in nursing homes is uncertain, it likely will have several features. Each episode of pressure ulcer development will be considered a learning experience; system factors contributing to the ulcer will be identified and corrected. A dedicated wound care team will exist to help institutionalize knowledge regarding best practices. This is preferred to a single wound care specialist, because too much knowledge may be lost if this person leaves the nursing home. Barriers to obtaining needed supplies, such as support surfaces, in a timely manner will be eliminated. Prompting systems to remind staff of the need to reposition patients will be in place. Above all, the nursing home must emphasize a culture of excellence in which quality care is routinely expected.

Achieving six-sigma quality in pressure ulcer care may not be possible; after all, health care is not the same as industrial production, but significant improvements are certainly achievable and worth striving for. Such improvements, though, will not be possible without better methods of assessing the quality of pressure ulcer care. This will be the challenge to researchers such as Bates-Jensen et al. One would hope that we could do better in pressure ulcer care than the airline industry does in handling our luggage.

---

[a] *From* Berlowitz D. Striving for six sigma in pressure ulcer care. J Am Geriatr Soc 2003;51:1320–1; with permission.

the 8-month follow-up showed that 55% of the nurses had implemented new pressure ulcer prevention routines. Documentation was still lacking after the program, although it was more detailed.

The nursing staff of a 500-bed Midwest U.S. hospital developed a pressure ulcer prevention program when the results of a quality improvement survey indicated both an increase in the number of pressure ulcers and a higher prevalence than the national average. Pressure ulcer incidence was used as the indicator of prevention strategy effectiveness. After a pressure ulcer education and incidence tracking mechanism was instituted, the affect of prevention measures increased, and most nursing units experienced a 10% to 20% decrease in the incidence of pressure ulcers [93].

An evidence-based education program for pressure ulcer prevention was conducted with a convenience sample of 59 registered and licensed practical nurses employed in three acute care hospitals [94]. The "Pressure Ulcer Knowledge" test was administered three times: immediately before (pre-test) and after (post-test 1) a standard pressure ulcer education workshop and again 3 months later (post-test 2). Registered nurses' knowledge scores were significantly higher than those of licensed practical nurses. Knowledge scores of the entire group were significantly higher from pre-test to post-test 1 and from pre-test to post-test 2 but significantly lower from post-test 1 to post-test 2, demonstrating that knowledge is not always retained over time.

Quality improvement

Halfens and Haalboom [10] reviewed pressure ulcer study publications from 1965 to 1999 using information available on Medline. Results showed that 0.06% of all Medline articles were related to pressure ulcers. Of all the articles about pressure ulcers, 49% were research articles, and 51% were clinical articles. The authors reported that the number and proportion of pressure ulcer articles are growing, as are initiatives urging researchers to start international working groups.

Hospital-acquired pressure ulcers continue to be a major quality management issue in which the estimates of prevalence and costs remain substantial and under-reported. Presently, 1.5 to 3 million patients with pressure ulcers require care at an approximate expense of $5 billion annually. More importantly, skin breakdown decreases the quality of life, thus adding to the burden of illness for patients and their caregivers. Moreover, pressure ulcers have been associated with in-hospital mortality. Allman et al [36] noted that hospitalized older adults with pressure ulcers are 2 times more likely to die within 30 days of discharge. Thomas et al [95] also noted that in-hospital pressure ulcers were associated with greater risk of death at 1 year after hospital discharge.

The absence or presence of pressure ulcers is used by the Health Care Financing Administration (now CMS) for survey and certification in long-term care as one benchmark of quality. MDS data [29] were used to evaluate a large provider of nursing home care to determine if there was improvement in the quality of care. Rates of pressure ulcer development were calculated for successive 6 month periods by determining the proportion of residents initially ulcer-free and having Stage II or greater on subsequent assessments. There was significant improvement in the quality of pressure ulcer preventive care from 1991–1995. These nursing homes showed a pressure ulcer rate decline of 25% and a decrease in the proportion of Stage III or IV ulcers. MDS data also have been used by researchers to derive a risk-adjustment model for pressure ulcer development that could be useful for profiling nursing homes on their rate of pressure ulcer development [30].

As nursing systems across the United States strive for Magnet Recognition Program status from the American Nurses Credentialing Center (ANCC), pressure ulcers will continue to surface as a quality of care issue. It is generally agreed that most pressure ulcers are avoidable. Nevertheless, despite an evolving mass of skin care research, the debate persists about the best practice to address the problem. As more evidence in the form of clinical practice guidelines becomes available to support quality programs, hospitals must identify and execute effective approaches to translate the information into practice. Regrettably, although the use of scientific evidence is heralded as the hallmark of practice, frontline clinicians often shift skin care to a low priority, particularly in tertiary care hospitals. Graham and Logan [96] describe the process of implementing an evidence-based skin care program in a surgical department of a large academic tertiary care hospital. The impetus to focus on skin care was the results from an annual prevalence survey that disclosed increasing rates and severity of ulcers for the in-patient surgical population. An interdisciplinary approach for the prevention and treatment of pressure ulcers was implemented.

In Canada, a survey [97] of the prevalence and incidence of pressure ulcers in two long-term care facilities was conducted on a single day. The incidence studies were completed 41 and 42 days later. Each resident was assessed for the presence and stage of pressure ulcers. The prevalence of pressure ulcers in the two long-term care facilities was 36.8% and 53.2%, respectively. The incidence of pressure ulcers in the two long-term care facilities was 11.7% and 11.6%, respectively. The authors claim that the pressure ulcer prevalence is higher than published figures for the long-term care setting. However, they believe that a pressure ulcer incidence of less than 12% in each facility suggests an equal and acceptable level of nursing care.

Nursing homes today face an increasing amount of oversight as they try to comply with regulations from federal, state, and local governments and agencies. Recent studies show that many facilities are not meeting basic quality of care guidelines for the prevention and treatment of pressure ulcers. Clinical practice guidelines disseminated by the AHRQ sought to improve clinical outcomes. These pressure ulcer guidelines were adapted by the American Medical Directors Association for use in long-term care. Unfortunately, the translation of the guideline recommendations into practice remains problematic. The trend of judicial oversight, particularly in cases involving pressure ulcers, presents a unique problem in pressure ulcer measurement. The Centers for Medicare and Medicaid Services considers a nosocomial Stage III or IV pressure ulcer as a sentinel event in a long-term care resident who has been assessed at low risk for pressure ulcers.

In 2002, Taler [82] asked what prevalence studies of pressure ulcers in nursing homes really tell us. He stated that pressure ulcers have long been considered emblematic of poor nursing care and have drawn the attention of many quality improvement initiatives, state and federal surveyors, and trial lawyers. He expressed his disappointment in the findings of Coleman et al [31] who showed that pressure ulcer prevalence had not changed since the implementation of the Omnibus Budget Reconciliation Act of 1987. He continues with a plea for better designed methods of collecting pressure ulcer data and explains there is an implicit assumption that a direct association exists between prevalence and incidence. This can lead to erroneous assumptions and there are important policy implications depending on the interpretation of pressure ulcer prevalence data.

Researchers from the University of Pennsylvania [98] studied data from 59 long-term care facilities in Maryland. Of the 2015 residents studied, 208 had one or more pressure ulcers on admission to a long-term care facility. The proportion of patients admitted from a hospital was 11.9% compared with 4.7% from those not admitted from a hospital. A lower prevalence of pressure ulcers on admission was significantly associated with being white. A higher prevalence on admission was associated with being bed- or chair-bound, underweight, and having fecal incontinence. Admission to a long-term care facility from a hospital is an important marker for a higher risk of pressure ulcers. The identification of risk factors is essential to the implementation of prevention activities [9,98].

The MDS is a comprehensive assessment tool for nursing home residents. The MDS 2.0 was used to obtain prevalence data from a hospital-based skilled nursing facility, and a survey was conducted to obtain skin care practices. The majority of residents were admitted from acute care facilities, and the prevalence of pressure ulcers was 18 ± 8.0%. Results were disappointing in that fundamental nursing routines such as toileting residents and keeping the head of the bed at an angle of less than 30° were not recognized as important interventions. Fewer than half of the facilities reported daily assessment and documentation of wound status. The investigators suggest that pressure ulcers are a common problem in acute care and hospital-based skilled nursing facilities. Research-based risk assessment, prevention, and wound care have not been widely implemented, and educational programs are needed [99].

The staff at 35 Veterans Affairs nursing homes was queried about quality improvement implementation activities, organizational culture, and their affect on pressure ulcer care. Completed surveys from 1065 nursing home staff members contained information on quality improvement, organization culture, employee satisfaction, and perceived adoption of pressure ulcer care guidelines. Data were compared with information abstracted from medical records. Quality improvement implementation was greater in nursing homes with an organizational culture that emphasized innovation and teamwork. Employees of nursing homes with a greater degree of quality improvement implementation were more satisfied with their jobs and were more likely to report adopting pressure ulcer clinical practice guidelines [100]. Researchers at a veterans' home in Iowa agreed with this finding and found the success of sustaining research-based pressure ulcer treatment protocols over a 5-year period provided evidence that the organizational culture of the facility and its department of nursing may be significant factors [101].

In America, the "Health Care Objectives for the Nation" report [102] includes an objective to "reduce the proportion of nursing home residents with current diagnosis of pressure ulcers" (http://www.healthypeople.gov). One of the National Quality Forum (NQF, available at: http://www.qualityforum.org) healthcare safety practices is the evaluation of patients for pressure ulcer risk. Monitoring patient risk status and performing therapeutic treatments are nursing functions that directly affect patient safety. Accomplishing these activities requires nursing staff with the clinical knowledge and skills needed to carry out preventive and therapeutic interventions. The Institute of Medicine report [27], "Keeping Patients

Safe," recommends maximizing the capability of the work force as a safety defense.

Summary

Pressure ulcers are a common and frustrating problem. Pressure ulcers increase demands on health care resources and are sometimes a source of malpractice litigation. Skin breakdown, often an iatrogenic complication of hospitalization, increases the length of stay and contributes to mortality and morbidity. Long-term care facilities are under increasing regulatory pressure to reduce rates of pressure ulcer occurrence [103]. The process-outcome link continues to escape us. Processes of care seem disjointed. Numerous studies [98–100,104,108] show a failure to implement what we know. When pressure ulcer risk is identified, preventive measures often are not implemented. The literature is replete with reports of quality improvement activities that enumerate multiple opportunities to improve care related to pressure ulcers [78,79,105–108]. Various quality improvement strategies for pressure ulcer prevention and management [109,110] have been produced, but recommendations are not always applied to practice [111]. When studies compared various outcomes before and after implementation of guidelines, most of the evidence was clinical audit data. Overall, active strategies were associated with better outcomes and passive strategies with poorer ones. Baier et al [112] reported improvement in processes of care after using a structured quality improvement approach in the long-term care setting [112,113]. Targeted education sessions were common to all studies reporting successful outcomes. Multidisciplinary wound care teams that conduct rounds at the bedside are highly recommended to enhance patient outcomes [114]. Functioning interdisciplinary teams clearly represent an important approach to error reduction [115]. To close the gap between risk identification and pressure ulcer prevention, we should develop active multidisciplinary wound care teams and "Strive for Six Sigma in Pressure Ulcer Care" [76].

References

[1] Petersen NC, Bittman S. The epidemiology of pressure sores. Scand J Plast Reconstr Surg 1971;5(1):62–6.
[2] Dinsdale SM. Decubitus ulcers: role of pressure and friction in causation. Arch Phys Med Rehab 1974;55:10–4.
[3] Daniel RK, Priest DI, Wheatley DC. Etiologic factors in pressure sores: an experimental model. Arch Phys Med Rehabil 1981;62:492–8.
[4] Allman RM. Pressure ulcers. In: Hazzard WR, Blass JP, Ettinger WH Jr, et al, editors. Principles of geriatric medicine and gerontology. 4th edition. New York: McGraw-Hill; 1999. p. 1577–83.
[5] Maklebust J. Pressure ulcers: etiology and prevention. Nurs Clin North Am 1987;22(2): 359–77.

[6] Panel for the Prediction and Prevention of Pressure Ulcers in Adults. Pressure ulcers in adults: prediction and prevention. [Clinical practice guideline No. 3.] Washington, DC: Agency for Health Care Policy and Research; 1992. US Department of Health and Human Services, AHCPR Publication # 92-0047.

[7] Bergstrom N, Bennett MA, Carlson CE, et al. Treatment of pressure ulcers. [Clinical practice guideline No. 15.] Rockville (MD): Agency for Health Care Policy and Research; 1994. US Dept of Health and Human Services, AHCPR Publication # 95-0652.

[8] Wound Ostomy Continence Nurses Society. Guideline for prevention and management of pressure ulcers. WOCN Clinical practice guideline series. Glenview (IL): WOCN; 2003.

[9] Thomas DR. Issues and dilemmas in the prevention and treatment of pressure ulcers: a review. J Gerontol A Biol Sci Med Sci 2001;56A:M328–40.

[10] Halfens R, Haalboom J. A historical overview of the pressure ulcer literature of the past 35 years. Ostomy Wound Manage 2001;47(11):36–43.

[11] Ankrom MA, Bennett RG, Sprigle S, et al. Pressure related deep tissue injury under intact skin and the current pressure ulcer staging systems. Advances in Skin and Wound Care 2005; (in press).

[12] Brandeis GH, Morris JN, Nash DJ. The epidemiology and natural history of pressure ulcers in elderly nursing home residents. JAMA 1990;(22):2905–9.

[13] National Pressure Ulcer Advisory Panel. Pressure ulcers, incidence, economics, risk assessment: consensus development conference statement. Decubitus 1989;2(2):24–8.

[14] Maklebust J. Perplexing questions about pressure ulcers. Decubitus 1992;5(7):15.

[15] Maklebust J. Pressure ulcer staging systems: intent, limitations, expectations. Adv Wound Care 1995;8(Suppl):S11–4.

[16] Maklebust J. Policy implications for using reverse staging to monitor pressure ulcer status. Adv Wound Care 1997;10(5):32–5.

[17] Glover D. Are pressure ulcers preventable: the debate is heating up. J Wound Care 2004; 13(3):83.

[18] Thomas DR. Are all pressure ulcers avoidable? J Am Med Dir Assoc 2001;2:297–301.

[19] Brandeis GH, Berlowitz D, Katz P. Are pressure ulcers preventable: a survey of experts. Adv Skin Wound Care 2001;14(5):244–8.

[20] Witkowsi J, Parish L. The decubitus ulcer: skin failure and destructive behavior. Int J Dermatol 2000;39:892–8.

[21] Ferrell B. Pressure ulcers: assessment of healing. Clin Geriatr Medicine 1997;18(13):575–86.

[22] Berlowitz D, Brandeis G, Anderson J, et al. Predictors of pressure ulcer healing among long-term care residents. J Am Geriatr Soc 1997;45(1):30–4.

[23] Brown G. Long-term outcomes of full-thickness pressure ulcers: healing and mortality. Ostomy Wound Manage 2003;49(10):42–50.

[24] Ennis WJ, Meneses P. Wound healing at the local level: the stunned wound. Ostomy Wound Manage 2000;46(Suppl 1A):S39–48.

[25] Ennis WJ. Healing: can we, must we, should we? Ostomy Wound Manage 2001;47(9):6–8.

[26] Kohn LT, Corrigan JM, Donaldson MS. To err is human: building a safer health system. Washington (DC): National Academy Press; 1999.

[27] Institute of Medicine. Keeping patients safe; priority areas for national action: transforming health care quality. Available at: http://www.iom.edu. Accessed October 20, 2004.

[28] McGlynn EA, Cassel CK, Leatherman ST, et al. Establishing national goals for quality improvement. Med Care 2003;41(Suppl 1):116–29.

[29] Brandeis GH, Berlowitz DR, Hossain M, et al. Pressure ulcers, the minimum data set and resident assessment protocol. Adv Wound Care 1995;8(6):18–25.

[30] Berlowitz DR, Brandesi GH, Morris JN, et al. Deriving a risk adjustment model for pressure ulcer development using the minimum data set. J Am Geriatr Soc 2001;49(7): 866–71.

[31] Coleman EA, Martau JM, Lim MK. Pressure ulcer prevalence in long term nursing home residents since the implementation of OBRA 1987. J Am Geriatr Soc 2002;50:728–32.

[32] Parish LC, Witkowski JT, Crissy JT. The decubitus ulcer in clinical practice. New York: Springer-Verlag; 1997.

[33] Versluysen M. Pressure sores in elderly patients: the epidemiology related to hip operations. J Bone Joint Surg Br 1985;7(1):10.

[34] Bliss M, Simini B. When are the seeds of postoperative pressure sores sown: often during surgery. BMJ 1999;319(7214):863–4.

[35] Schoonhoven L, Defloor T, van der Tweel I, et al. Risk indicators for pressure ulcers during surgery. Appl Nurs Res 2002;16(2):163–73.

[36] Allman RM, Laprade CA, Noel LB, et al. Pressure sores among hospitalized patients. Ann Intern Med 1986;105(3):337.

[37] Thomas DR, Allman R, editors. Pressure ulcers. Clinics in Geriatric Medicine 1997; 13(3):13.

[38] Maklebust J, Sieggreen M. Pressure ulcers: guidelines for prevention and management. 3rd edition. Springhouse (PA): Springhouse Corporation; 2001.

[39] Pieper B. Mechanical forces: pressure, shear, and friction in acute and chronic wounds, nursing management. In: Bryant R, editor. 2nd edition. St Louis (MO): Mosby; 2000.

[40] Krasner D, Rodeheaver GT, Sibbald RG. Chronic wound care: a clinical source book for healthcare professionals. 3rd edition. Wayne (PA): HMP Communications; 2001.

[41] Baranoski S, Ayello EA. Wound care essentials: practice principles. Philadelphia: Lippincott Williams & Wilkins; 2004.

[42] Cuddigan J, Berlowitz DR, Ayello EA, editors. Pressure ulcers in America: prevalence, incidence, and implications for the future. National Pressure Ulcer Advisory Panel Monograph. Reston (VA): NPUAP; 2001.

[43] Salzberg CA, Byrne DW, Cayten CG, et al. Predicting and preventing pressure ulcers in adults with paralysis. Adv Wound Care 1998;11(5):237–46.

[44] Meehan M. National pressure ulcer prevalence survey. Adv Wound Care 1994;7:27–30, 34, 36–8.

[45] Ayello EA, Lyder CH. Pressure ulcers in persons of color, race, and ethnicity. In: Cuddigan J, editor. Pressure ulcers in America: prevalence, incidence and implications for the future. Washington (DC): National Pressure Ulcer Advisory Panel; 2001. p. 153–62.

[46] Shea JD. Pressure sores: classification and management. Clin Orthop 1975;112:89–100.

[47] Lyder CH. Examining the inclusion of ethnic minorities in pressure ulcer prediction studies. J Wound Ostomy Continence Nurs 1996;23:257–60.

[48] Henderson C, Ayello E, Sussman C, et al. Draft definition of stage I pressure ulcers: inclusion of persons with darkly pigmented skin. Adv Wound Care 1997;10(5):16–9.

[49] Matas A, Sowa M, Taylor V, et al. Eliminating the issue of skin color in assessment of the blanch response. Adv Skin Wound Care 2001;14(4):180–8.

[50] Sprigle S, Linden M, McKenna D, et al. Clinical skin temperature measurement to predict incipient pressure ulcers. Adv Skin Wound Care 2001;114(3):133–7.

[51] Bethell E. Controversies in classifying and assessing grade I pressure ulcers. J Wound Care 2003;12(1):33.

[52] Ayello EA, Braden BJ. How and why to do pressure ulcer risk assessment. Adv Wound Care 2002;15(3):125–31.

[53] American Medical Directors Association. Pressure ulcer therapy companion: clinical practice guideline. Columbia (MD): AMDA; 1999.

[54] Braden BJ, Bergstrom NA. Clinical utility of the Braden scale for predicting pressure sore risk. Decubitus 1989;2(3):44–51.

[55] Bergstrom NA, Braden BJ. A prospective study of pressure sore risk among institutionalized elderly. J Am Geriatr Soc 1992;40:747–58.

[56] Bergstrom NA, Braden BJ, Kemp M, et al. Multi-site study of the incidence of pressure ulcers and the relationship between risk level, demographic characteristics, diagnoses, and prescription of preventive interventions. J Am Geriatr Soc 1996;44:22–30.

[57] Bergstrom NA. Predicting pressure ulcer risk: a multisite study of the predictive validity of the Braden Scale. Nurs Res 1998;47(5):261–9.

[58] Lyder CH. Validating the Braden Scale for the prediction of pressure ulcer risk in blacks and Latino/Hispanic elders: a pilot study. Ostomy Wound Manage 1998;44(3A):42.

[59] Berquist S. Subscales, subscores, or summative score; evaluating the contribution of Braden Scale items for predicting pressure ulcer risk in older adults receiving home health care. J Wound Ostomy Continence Nurs 2001;28:279–89.

[60] Bergquist S, Frantz R. Braden Scale: Validity in community-based older adult receiving home health care. Appl Nurs Res 2001;14(1):36–43.

[61] Ramundo JM. Reliability and validity of the Braden Scale in the home care setting. J Wound Ostomy Continence Nurs 1995;21(1):128–34.

[62] Bergstrom NA. Strategies for preventing pressure ulcers. Clin Geriatr Med 1997;13(3):437–54.

[63] Lyder CH. Pressure ulcer prevention and management. JAMA 2003;289(2):223–6.

[64] Hergenroeder P, Mosher C, Sevo D. Pressure ulcer risk assessment: simple or complex? Decubitus 1992;5(7):47–8, 50–2.

[65] Salvadina GD, Snyder ML, Brogdon KE. Clinical trial of the Braden Scale on an acute care medical unit. J Enterostomal Ther 1992;19:160–5.

[66] Maklebust J, Sieggreen M, Sidor D, et al. Computer-based testing of the Braden Scale for predicting pressure sore risk. Ostomy Wound Manage 2005; in press.

[67] Thomas DR. Prevention and treatment of pressure ulcers: what works, what doesn't? Cleve Clin J Med 2001;68(8):704–22.

[68] Fisher AR, Wells G, Harrison MB. Factors associated with pressure ulcers in adults in acute care hospitals. Adv Skin Wound Care 2004;17(2):80–90.

[69] Olshansky K. Pressure ulcer prevention: where did we go wrong? Ostomy Wound Manage 2004;3(3):6–8.

[70] National Pressure Ulcer Advisory Panel position statement on reverse staging of pressure ulcers. Available at: http://www.npuap.org. Accessed October 20, 2004.

[71] Bates-Jensen BM. The pressure sore status tool a few thousand assessments later. Adv Wound Care 1997;10(5):65–73.

[72] Thomas DR, Rodeheaver GT, Bartolucci AA, et al. The pressure ulcer scale for healing: derivation and validation of the PUSH tool. Adv Wound Care 1997;10(5):96–101.

[73] Ferrell BA. The Sessing scale for measurement of pressure ulcer healing. Adv Wound Care 1997;10(5):78–80.

[74] Krasner D. Wound healing scale, version 1.0: a proposal. Adv Wound Care 1997;1(5):82–5.

[75] Stotts N, Rodeheaver G, Thomas D, et al. An instrument to measure healing in pressure ulcers: development and validation of the pressure ulcer scale for healing (PUSH). J Gerontol 2001;56A(12):M795–9.

[76] Berlowitz D. Striving for six sigma in pressure ulcer care. J Am Geriatr Soc 2003;51:1320–1.

[77] Chassin MR. Is health care ready for six sigma quality? Milbank Q 1998;76:565–91.

[78] Bates-Jensen BM, Cadogan M, Jorge J, et al. Standardized quality assessment system to evaluate pressure ulcer care in the nursing home. J Am Geriatr Soc 2003;51:1194–201.

[79] Bates-Jensen BM, Cadogan M, Osterweil D, et al. The minimum data set pressure ulcer indicator: does it reflect differences in care processes related to pressure ulcer prevention and treatment in nursing homes? J Am Geriatr Soc 2003;51:1202–11.

[80] Saliba D, Rubenstein LV, Simon B, et al. Adherence to pressure ulcer prevention guidelines: implications for nursing home quality. J Am Geriatr Soc 2003;51:56–62.

[81] Kane RL. Assuring quality in nursing home care. J Am Geriatr Soc 1998;46:232–7.

[82] Taler G. What do prevalence studies of pressure ulcers in nursing homes really tell us? J Am Geriatr Soc 2002;50:773–4.

[83] Xakellis GC, Frantz RA, Lewis A, et al. Translating pressure ulcer guidelines into practice: it's harder than it sounds. Adv Skin Wound Care 2001;14(5):249–56.

[84] Young Z, Evans A, Davis J. Clinical issues: nosocomial pressure ulcer prevention: a successful project. JONA 2003;33(7/8):380–3.

[85] Pieper B, Sugrue M, Weiland M, et al. Presence of pressure ulcer prevention methods used among patients considered at risk versus those considered not at risk. J Wound Ostomy Continence Nurs 1997;24(4):191–9.

[86] Pieper B, Mott M. Nurses knowledge of pressure ulcer prevention, staging and description. Adv Wound Care 1995;8(3):34.

[87] Vogelpohl T, Doughety J. What do nursing students learn about pressure ulcers: survey of content on pressure ulcers in nursing school textbooks. Decubitus 1993;6:48–52.

[88] Ayello E, Meaney G. Replicating a survey of pressure ulcer content in nursing textbooks. J Wound Ostomy Continence Nurs 2003;30:266–71.

[89] Odierna E, Zeleznik J. Pressure ulcer education: a pilot study of the knowledge and clinical confidence of geriatric fellows. Adv Skin Wound Care 2003;16(1):26–30.

[90] Lyder CH. Pressure ulcers. In: Cobbs EL, Duthie EH Jr, Murphy JB, editors. Geriatrics review syllabus: a core curriculum in geriatric medicine. 5th edition. Malden (MA): Blackwell; 2002. p. 202–9.

[91] Caliri M, Miyazaki M, Pieper B. Knowledge of pressure ulcers by undergraduate nursing students in Brazil. Ostomy Wound Manage 2002;49(3):54–63.

[92] Gunningberg L. Pressure ulcer prevention: evaluation of an education program for Swedish nurses. J Wound Care 2004;13(3):85.

[93] Robinson C, Gloeckner M, Bush S, et al. Determining the efficacy of a pressure ulcer prevention program by collecting prevalence and incidence data: a unit-based effort. Ostomy Wound Manage 2003;49(5):44–51.

[94] Sinclair L, Berwiczonek H, Thurston N, et al. Evaluation of an evidence-based education program for pressure ulcer prevention. J Wound Ostomy Continence Nurs 2004;31(1): 43–50.

[95] Thomas DR, Goode PS, Tarquine PH, et al. Hospital acquired pressure ulcers and risk of death. J Am Geriatr Soc 1996;44:1435–40.

[96] Graham K, Logan J. Using the Ottawa model of research use to implement a skin care program. J Nurs Care Qual 2004;19(1):18–26.

[97] Davis C, Caseby N. Prevalence and incidence studies of pressure ulcers in two long-term care facilities in Canada. Ostomy Wound Manage 2001;47(11):28–34.

[98] Baumgarten M, Margolis D, Gruber-Baldini AL, et al. Pressure ulcers and the transition to long-term care. Adv Skin Wound Care 2003;16(6):299–304.

[99] Siem C, Wipke-Tevis D, Rantz M, et al. Skin assessment and pressure ulcer based care in hospital-based skilled nursing facilities. Ostomy Wound Manage 2003;49(6):42–58.

[100] Berlowitz D, Young G, Hickey E, et al. Quality improvement implementation in the nursing home. Health Serv Res 2003;38:65–83.

[101] America: the health care objectives for the nation: healthy people 2010. Available at: http:// www.healthypeople.gov. Accessed October 20, 2004.

[102] Bates-Jensen BM. Quality indicators for prevention and management of pressure ulcers in vulnerable elders. Ann Intern Med 2001;135:744–51.

[103] Spector WD. Correlates of pressure sores in nursing homes: evidence from the National Medical Expenditure Survey. J Invest Dermatol 1994;102:42S–5S.

[104] Frantz F, Gardner S, Specht J, et al. Integration of pressure ulcer treatment protocol into practice: clinical outcomes and care environment attributes. Outcomes Management 2001; 5(3):112–20.

[105] Harrison MB, Logan J, Joseph L, et al. Quality improvement, research and evidence-based practice: five years experience with pressure ulcers. Evid Based Nurs 1998;1:108–10.

[106] Lyder CH, Preston J, Grady J, et al. Quality of care for hospitalized medicare patients at risk for pressure ulcers. Arch Intern Med 2001;161:1549–54.

[107] Xakellis GC. Quality assurance programs for pressure ulcers. Clin Geriatr Med 1997;13: 599–606.

[108] Allman RM. Pressure ulcers: using what we know to improve quality of care. J Am Geriatr Soc 2001;49:996–7.

[109] Bryant RA, Rolstad S. Utilizing a systems approach to implement pressure ulcer prediction and prevention. Ostomy Wound Manage 2001;47(9):26–36.

[110] Beitz JM. Overcoming barriers to quality wound care: a systems perspective. Ostomy Wound Manage 2001;47(3):56–64.

[111] Rutledge DN, Donaldson NE, Pravikoff DS. Protection of skin integrity: progress in pressure ulcer prevention since the AHCPR 1992 guideline. Online Journal of Clinical Innovations 2000;3(5):1–67.

[112] Baier RR, Gifford DR, Lyder CH, et al. Quality improvement for pressure ulcer care in the nursing home setting: the Northeast Pressure Ulcer Project. J Am Med Dir Assoc 2003;4: 291–301.

[113] Tooher R, Middleton P, Babidge W. Implementation of pressure ulcer guidelines: what constitutes a successful strategy? J Wound Care 2003;12(10):378.

[114] Trumner A, Panfil EM. Wound care teams for preventing and treating pressure ulcers (protocol for a Cochrane review). The Cochrane Library. Issue 4. Chichester (UK): John Wiley & Sons, Ltd.; 2003.

[115] Morley J, Flaherty J, Thomas DR. Geriatricians, continuous quality improvement and improved care for older people. J Gerontol 2003;58A(9):809–12.

ELSEVIER
SAUNDERS

Nurs Clin N Am 40 (2005) 391–410

NURSING
CLINICS
OF NORTH AMERICA

Lower Extremity Arterial and Venous Ulcers

Mary Sieggreen, MSN, APRN, CVN[a,b]

[a]Department of Vascular Surgery, Harper University Hospital,
Detroit Medical Center, Detroit, MI, USA
[b]Wayne State University College of Nursing, Detroit, MI, USA

The lower extremity ulcer is a common problem that results from many different clinical causes. Peripheral arterial disease affects 8 to 12 million individuals in the United States [1], and the incidence continues to rise annually [2,3]. Studies [4–8] of lower extremity ulcers report a prevalence ranging from 0.12% to 2.5% in the general and geriatric populations. The majority of patients with leg ulcers are elderly [5,9], and venous ulcers can be expected to increase as the mean age of the population increases. The most frequent cause for a leg ulcer is peripheral arterial or venous disease, although there can be mixed pathology. Management of these ulcers is complex and expensive. One study [10] reported that the annual cost to treat a venous ulcer ranges from $20,041 to $27,493 depending on the treatment. The treatment strategy requires an understanding of the underlying disease process as well as wound care. There are different types of vascular diseases, and each type has a different pathologic reason for ulcer development; treatment for one type may be detrimental to another. Noninvasive and invasive diagnostic studies are performed to identify wound cause and to determine the best course of treatment. Surgical intervention is frequently required to restore blood flow to the tissues, and careful medical management is necessary for coexisting diseases. Patients are expected to change life style routines and to give up habits that aggravate the disease process and contribute to ulcer formation or inhibit healing. There is considerable suffering and changes in quality of life for patients with chronic leg ulcers [11–13].

E-mail address: msieggre@dmc.org

Arterial and venous anatomy of the lower extremity

Arterial anatomy

It is useful to review arterial anatomy when considering arterial perfusion. Major arteries in the lower extremity are illustrated in Fig. 1. In reference to the lower extremities, arterial blood flow exits the heart and moves into the thoracic aorta and to the abdominal aorta, the common, internal and external iliac arteries, the common and internal and external femoral arteries, the popliteal, the anterior and posterior tibial and peroneal arteries and extends to the pedal arch.

Venous anatomy

The major veins are illustrated in Fig. 2. There are three systems of veins in the leg: the superficial, deep, and perforating veins. Each of these systems has valves that ensure unidirectional blood flow from the superficial through the perforators and into the deep system. Venous return to the heart is

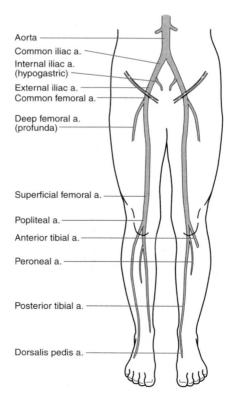

Fig. 1. Arterial anatomy of the lower extremities.

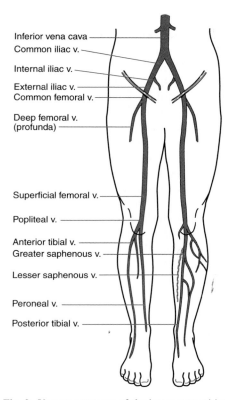

Inferior vena cava
Common iliac v.
Internal iliac v.
External iliac v.
Common femoral v.
Deep femoral v.
(profunda)
Superficial femoral v.
Popliteal v.
Anterior tibial v.
Greater saphenous v.
Lesser saphenous v.
Peroneal v.
Posterior tibial v.

Fig. 2. Venous anatomy of the lower extremities.

assisted by calf muscle contraction and pressure variation in the abdomen and thorax. Venous valves are bileaflets with valve sinuses at the base. With retrograde flow, the sinuses fill, and one leaflet stretches to meet the opposite one, closing the vein. Venous insufficiency occurs with the loss of valve function. Loss may be caused by a thrombus fixing the valve open or a weak and distended vein wall stretching so that the cusps do not meet. Either way, the blood will reflux distally, causing venous hypertension.

History and physical examination

Patients present to the vascular clinician with a leg ulcer for one of three reasons: progressive pain, a nonhealing wound, or a vascular disease diagnosed by the patient's primary care provider. Patients seek medical care for an ischemic ulcer most commonly because of pain, whereas they seek treatment for a venous ulcer because of drainage or swelling. When obtaining a history, caregivers should inquire whether claudication was present before the ulcer developed. Claudication is pain in the calf muscle, which occurs when walking a predictable distance, and is relieved when ambulation is stopped. If another problem is causing the pain, cessation of ambulation will not provide relief. Claudication may occur in the calves, thighs, or buttocks depending on the location of the arterial lesion. When taking a history from a patient with other conditions that may inhibit walking, the patient may not be able to ambulate far enough to elicit claudication symptoms; denial of leg pain from a nonambulating patient does not exclude arterial disease.

As arterial disease becomes worse, pain may be in the foot or toes at night, waking the patient from sleep. Blood pressure is lowered during sleep, and the pressure may not be sufficient to oxygenate the tissues of the foot, causing ischemic pain, also described as "rest pain." Patients relieve this pain by placing the leg in a dependant position, using gravity to enhance flow to the foot. Patients with diabetes may not experience this pain in the presence of severe neuropathy. Rest pain with or without ulcers requires immediate restoration of blood flow in an attempt to prevent amputation of the affected limb.

Physical examination

Inspection

Assessment of a patient presenting with a leg ulcer includes a general physical examination with special focus on the vascular system. Visual examination of the skin provides an indication of the underlying vascular disease. Skin color may indicate perfusion problems in the arterial or venous system. Ischemic tissue initially appears pale compared with the rest of the patient's skin. When tissue oxygenation decreases, the skin takes on a mottled appearance and becomes darker as the tissue dies. Patients with chronic arterial insufficiency may have thin, pale, shiny, hairless skin, and thickened nails; however these are not reliable signs of ischemia. Thick nails are caused by other underlying problems, most often fungal infections. Acute arterial disease will not have any of the chronic skin changes. Ischemic limbs demonstrate a characteristic pallor when elevated to 45°. When placed in the dependant position after elevation, the skin changes to a deep reddish color as the foot fills with blood; this is called dependant rubor. This is a pathopneumonic response in ischemic tissue. Capillary refill, another test of skin perfusion, is checked by placing pressure against the toe pad until it becomes pale, and the time it takes to return to a normal color is measured. A capillary refill time longer than 3 seconds indicates decreased perfusion.

Skin color changes resulting from venous disease range from a bluish purple, caused by engorged veins, to a darkened brownish rusty color of the skin in advanced venous disease. The color appears in the gaitor area from the ankles to approximately mid calf. Ankle edema is present in venous insufficiency. In longstanding venous disease, the skin and underlying tissue may have lipodermatosclerosis, a condition of fibrotic skin, and underlying tissue that is not well oxygenated. It does not have the elasticity of healthy tissue and will not expand with increased fluid accumulation. Frequent tissue breakdown and healing problems are common in this area.

Palpation

The skin is palpated for temperature. An ischemic leg is cooler to palpation than the opposite leg or the more proximal part of the same leg if it is not involved in the ischemia. The leg with venous insufficiency may be warmer than the contralateral leg or the more proximal tissue. Palpating all pulses and comparing contralateral pulses is one of the most important parts of the examination. Pulses may be absent or diminished in the limb with an arterial ulcer, or they may not be palpable in the presence of venous disease caused by edema. Patients with claudication may have palpable pulses while sitting in the examination room only to have them disappear when ambulating to the point of claudication. The dorsalis pedis pulse is congenitally absent in 10% of individuals.

Blood pressure and the ankle brachial index

Blood pressure is measured in all extremities. A systolic pressure difference of 20 mm Hg between contralateral extremities or between segmental pressures in the same limb indicates proximal arterial stenosis. An ankle brachial index (ABI) is used to assess arterial disease in the lower extremities. This test is performed using a blood pressure cuff and a handheld Doppler ultrasonogram transducer. The patient should be in a supine position for approximately 10 minutes. Bilateral brachial blood pressure measurements are obtained. The higher of the two systolic pressures is used as the denominator. A blood pressure cuff is placed around the leg above the ankle. The dorsalis pedis or posterior tibial artery is identified by palpation. After placing the transducer gel on the skin, the Doppler probe is placed over one of these arteries. The blood pressure cuff is inflated and carefully deflated until a sound is heard. This is the ankle systolic pressure, which becomes the numerator. The ankle pressure is divided by the brachial pressure to obtain the ABI. The ABI is interpreted in light of the patient's symptoms. If the ABI is greater than 1.0 in a diabetic patient, it is falsely high. In this patient population toe brachial index (TBI) are more accurate and should be obtained instead of an ABI. See Box 1 for ABI interpretation.

A problem associated with leg ulcers is decreased sensory perception in patients with diabetes. This is best tested by gently placing the tip of the Semmes-Weinstein monofilament against the tissue to be tested. When the filament bends, the patient with normal sensation should be able to feel the pressure.

Box 1. ABI and arterial disease

0.9 to 1.0 = normal
0.89 to 0.6 = mild disease (the patient may be without symptoms)
0.59 to 0.4 = moderate disease (the patient may have symptoms,
     and wounds may not heal)
below 0.4 = severe disease (the patient experiences rest pain;
     wounds will not heal)
more than 1.0 consider vessel calcification

Vascular testing

The first priority is to determine arterial inflow status. This is done by performing noninvasive tests in the vascular laboratory and contrast arteriograms in the radiology suite. Based on these tests, arterial flow and patency are determined; and based on the findings, an operation or a percutaneous procedure may be recommended.

Noninvasive tests performed in the vascular laboratory provide dynamic information about vascular function. Arterial tests include Doppler ultrasonography, segmental pressures, and waveforms. Venous studies include ultrasonography to determine old or new deep vein thrombosis, and a venous duplex is performed to assess valve function. Transcutaneous oxygen pressure can also be measured in the vascular laboratory. An invasive arteriogram is performed only if a patient is willing to undergo an operative or percutaneous procedure.

Arterial ulcer

Arterial ulcers occur when the arterial blood supply cannot meet the metabolic tissue needs. Arterial insufficiency may affect any part of the body but is found most frequently in the lower extremities. Tips of the fingers may be affected in the presence of vasospastic and rheumatologic vasculitic disorders, but lower extremity ulcers are most likely to be the result of atherosclerosis. The precipitating event causing an ulcer might be a minor trauma in the presence of underlying vascular disease. A wound that does not heal may be the first indication of arterial or venous insufficiency.

Acute limb ischemia can also cause arterial ulceration. Most acute ischemia has underlying atherosclerosis but the ulcer can be caused by a thrombosis or embolus. This situation is precipitated by an acute event or a chronic condition. A thrombus can originate from an atherosclerotic plaque or an occluded surgical bypass graft. An embolism can be part of a plaque or a platelet thrombus that breaks away from its origin, which could be any proximal site, including the heart. The embolism obstructs a more distal artery, effectively stopping flow to the tissues. Other

nonatherosclerotic diseases such as arterial trauma, arteritis, and hyperco-
agulable disorders can cause acute ischemia (Fig. 3).

Pathophysiology

Atherosclerosis is a chronic progressive disease involving arterial wall
thickening, which develops as a result of deposits of cellular debris including
lipids, platelets, and fibrin. The condition begins early in life with fatty
streaks deposited in the arterial wall that are believed to be reversible in this
early phase. Multiple factors contribute over time to increasing plaque
development. Symptoms usually appear sometime after the fourth decade of
life. An injury to the intimal lining stimulates platelet adhesiveness and
macrophage migration. Growth factors are released, which encourages
vascular smooth muscle cell proliferation. Plaque may extend into the media
of the wall causing vessel ulceration, with lipid and platelet deposit. Platelet
deposition continues in response to increased vessel wall injury. As the
plaque grows, the vessel lumen progressively narrows until blood flow is
affected. Common sites for plaque development are the aorta, bifurcations
to the iliac arteries, the common to the internal and external iliac arteries,
the common femoral bifurcation, and the superficial femoral artery at
Hunter's canal. The superficial femoral artery is the most commonly
occluded artery in the leg and is frequently responsible for lower leg
ischemia.

Ulcer characteristics

The base of an arterial ulcer is pale and dry. There may be a yellow
fibrotic film across the surface or, if this has dried, a black eschar. There
is no drainage or inflammation unless the ulcer is infected. The margins

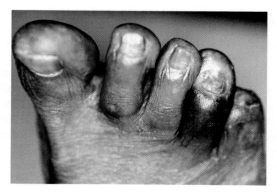

Fig. 3. Fourth and fifth toes are necrotic from atherosclerotic emboli showering into small
arteries.

are usually distinct. Nondiabetic patients describe ulcer pain as sharp, throbbing, or burning. Diabetic patients with neuropathy may report no pain, or they experience pain much later than the nondiabetic. Ischemic pain can become excruciating and may require appropriately large doses of narcotics for pain management. Pain is aggravated with dressing changes and wound manipulation. Arterial ulcers may remain stable with a progressive increase in pain as the tissue becomes more ischemic. As the tissue becomes mummified, the pain is felt at the line of demarcation.

Venous Ulcer

Patients with venous ulcers present with aching of the affected limb and edema that is more pronounced at the end of the day. Despite the common misconception that venous ulcers do not cause pain, up to 75% of patients with venous ulcers report that the discomfort is significant enough to interfere with their quality of life [14]. The venous ulcer is most commonly found above or around the medial malleolus and is shallow and has irregular borders. The size of the ulcers can range from very small to very large, completely encircling the leg, and edema is often present. There may be eczematous changes in the skin, varicose veins, and pigmentation. Patients may or may not describe a history of deep vein thrombosis, trauma, or a surgical procedure to the legs, groin, abdomen, or multiple pregnancies. Patients with longstanding lower extremity venous disease may have lipodermatosclerosis, a progressive fibrosing, inflammatory process of the dermis and subcutaneous tissue [15]. Risk factors identified in nonhealing venous ulcers despite appropriate treatment include a large wound area, duration of the wound, a history of vein ligation and hip or knee surgery, an ABI less than 0.80, and the presence of fibrin on more than 50% of the wound surface [16].

Pathophysiology

Venous hypertension is believed to play a significant role in the cause of venous ulcers. Deep, superficial, and perforator venous insufficiency resulting from incompetent valves causes venous hypertension (Fig. 4). High venous pressure in the capillary bed leads to vessel wall damage and loss of fluid into the interstitial space. This causes edema in the soft tissue of the ankle, the most dependent part of the leg. Fluid escape into the tissue is followed by red blood cells. The natural decomposition of red blood cells releasing hemosiderin creates the characteristic brown skin staining of the ankles in patients with longstanding venous disease. In addition to changes in skin color, the chronic fluid deposition creates fibrosis of the soft tissues, making them more vulnerable to trauma and less receptive to cellular oxygen transport. With an increase in fluid accumulation and maximal

Competent Venous Valves

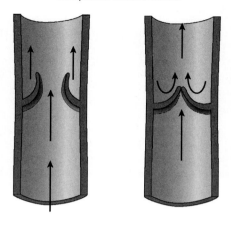

Incompetent Venous Valves

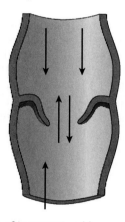

Fig. 4. Comparison of competent and incompetent venous valves.

stretching, the tissues begin to ooze or frankly open into a sore that becomes the venous ulcer (Fig. 5).

In an attempt to explain this phenomenon, several theories have been put forth. The most current are the "fibrin cuff" and the "white cell trapping" theories. The fibrin cuff theory [17] states that layers of fibrin are laid down around the capillary wall, causing a diffusion barrier to oxygen and nutrients. A variation of this theory is that there is a leakage of fibrinogen and protein-bound growth factors that are trapped in the pericapillary fibrin cuff, which prevents their use in tissue repair. The white cell trapping theory states that patients with venous hypertension accumulate neutrophils in the microcirculation, which produces toxic metabolites that lead to

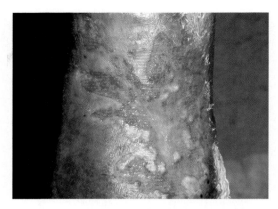

Fig. 5. The typical venous ulcer is shallow with irregular borders and new islands of epithelial growth.

lipodermatosclerosis. Increasing pressure reduces capillary perfusion pressure and flow rate, which leads to white blood cell adherence to the cell wall. Proteolytic enzymes, oxygen free radicals, and lipid products are released by the interaction of endothelial cells and leucocytes. The white cell activation damages cell walls, thereby increasing permeability and allowing larger molecules to get through the capillary walls [18].

These tissue changes make the skin more vulnerable to injury. There may be excoriation and pruritus. The skin may present as erythematous and weeping or with dry crusts. Frequently, patients have been instructed by other health care personnel or well-meaning friends and family members to use topical treatments that actually further exacerbate the dermatitis surrounding the leg ulcer [19].

Classification of venous disease

The American Venous Forum developed a classification system in 1994 for chronic venous disease that addresses the key elements in venous abnormalities. This classification system is based on clinical, causation, anatomic, and pathophysiologic data and is known as the Clinical Etiologic Anatomic Pathiophysiologic (CEAP) system [20]. The system is used to provide objective information about venous disease and clarify relationships among contributing factors. It provides a language that can be used to compare studies. The clinical classification subdivides ulcers into seven classes based on objective signs: class 0, no visible or palpable signs; class 1, telangiectasia; class 2, varicose veins; class 3, edema; class 4, skin changes, including pigmentation, eczema, lipodermatosclerosis; class 5, skin changes and a healed ulcer; and class 6, skin changes and an active ulcer. Each class is accompanied by a subscript letter A, meaning asymptomatic, or S, meaning symptomatic. Cause is divided into congenital, primary, or secondary. Anatomic classification, denoted by a lower-case letter, includes superficial (s), deep (d), and perforator veins (p). Pathophysiologic classification, denoted by a capital letter, is divided into reflux (R), obstruction (O), or both (R, O). The classification system is useful for communication among practitioners and allows the results of research studies to be compared. The practical advantage is that the classification score can direct the level of workup for each individual [21].

Risk factors for arterial ulcers

Associated conditions that aggravate the disease process or interfere with ulcer healing found frequently in patients with vascular disease include diabetes and renal disease. Individuals with diabetes are more likely to have peripheral arterial disease and a more rapid progression of the disease process than those who do not have diabetes. Other noncontrollable factors associated with vascular ulcers are a family history positive for atherosclerosis, age, and gender. Controllable risk factors for developing atherosclerosis include smoking, hyperlipidemia, hypertension, stress, a sedentary life style, and obesity (Box 2).

It is estimated that approximately 90% of patients with atherosclerosis are smokers. Nicotine and carbon monoxide in cigarettes are atherogenic components. Nicotine affects the sympathetic nervous system by constricting the wall of the arteries, and carbon monoxide binds with the hemoglobin molecule in preference to oxygen. Oxygen transport to the tissues is decreased. Smoking accelerates atherosclerosis postoperatively by the formation of myointimal hyperplasia. Smoking cessation has been shown to reduce peripheral arterial occlusive disease progression and improve maximal walking times [22]. Individuals with hypertension have a greater propensity to atherosclerotic disease than normotensive individuals. It is believed that the arterial intima is damaged with sustained high pressures.

Box 2. Risk factors

Age
Diabetes mellitus
Exercise
Family history
Gender
Hyperlipidemia
Hypertension
Smoking
Stress

Treatment for arterial ulcers

Treatment for arterial ulcers includes treatment of the arterial inflow problem that reduces blood flow to the leg. This approach most often requires an invasive procedure such as a percutaneous endovascular procedure or an open surgical repair.

Surgical procedures: revascularization

The standard treatment for ischemic ulcers is to restore blood flow by a surgical bypass procedure using a prosthetic graft or autogenous vein. Autogenous veins may be in situ or reversed veins [23]. The most common surgical operations are aorto-iliac bypass, femoral-popliteal bypass, and distal bypasses to the ankle or foot. The most proximal lesion is repaired first. If this is not sufficient to heal the ulcer, more distal arterial procedures are performed. Percutaneous procedures, which are most effective for short lesions in large vessels, include balloon dilation or stent placement. Open bypass operations have withstood the test of time, and all new procedures are compared with them for durability. When surgical options are chosen, the most proximal arterial lesion is treated first because this may be all that is needed to restore flow to heal the ulcer.

No surgical treatment

Medical treatment for arterial ulcers is limited. Treatment of the underlying disease process continues for life, including risk factor management and changes in lifestyle [24], smoking cessation [22], lipid management, maintaining an exercise program, and controlling hypertension are activities to reduce disease progression. One of the more promising medications, cilostazol (Pletal), from a new category of drugs called phosphodiesterase inhibitors, acts as a vasodilator and suppresses platelet aggregation. This drug is used for claudication [25,26]; however, improvement in arterial ulcer healing has been reported by one study [27]. With all the appropriate care provided for patients presenting with ischemic ulcers, patients whose ulcers showed no appreciable healing were given cilostazol. Approximately two thirds of the patients progressed to satisfactory healing after being placed on the drug. This was not a research study, but clearly there are possibilities for medical intervention that need to be tested further. Clinical trials are currently underway to test angiogenic growth factors as treatment modalities.

Researchers have shown that intermittent pneumatic compression is effective in stimulating blood flow in the treatment of arterial disease. A device consisting of a pump and cuff (the Art Assist), which fits over the foot and leg up to the knee, is applied to the leg. A pressure of 120 mm Hg is applied sequentially from the foot to the leg in a 3-cycle/minute schedule to simulate ambulation. Compression is used to empty the veins, thereby increasing the arterial venous pressure gradient that increases flow into the arteries. Noninvasive studies [28–30] have documented an increase in blood flow from 13% to 240% to the calf with this device. One study [31] reported complete healing in 25 patients who had no other option but amputation. Intermittent pneumatic compression, although tested in small studies, shows promise in improving blood flow and preventing amputation for selected patients who are not candidates for surgical reconstruction [32].

Treatment for venous ulcer

Compression

Compression is the mainstay of treatment for venous ulcers, and almost all lower-extremity venous disease [33,34]. It works by compressing the veins, restoring valvular competence, reducing venous hypertension in the legs, and minimizing edema [35]. Compression is delivered by elastic or non-elastic dressings applied with tension against the body surface to transmit pressure to the underlying tissue. It is used to counteract the venous hyper-tension in the leg, reduce edema, support the ulcer during healing, and to prevent the long term sequelae of venous disease (Box 3).

The difference between elastic and nonelastic material is that the elastic compression will change with the volume changes in the leg and continue to

---

Box 3. Products used to provide support and reduce edema

Nonelastic
CircAid Thera-boot
Gelocast
Tenderwrap Unna boot
UNNA-FLEX elastic Unna boot

Elastic
DYNA-FLEX cohesive compression bandage
SetoPress high compression bandage
SurePress high compression bandage
Profore four-layer bandage system

Therapeutic compression stocking manufacturers
Jobst, Box 471048, Charlotte, NC 28247; 800-537-1063;
    www.Jobst-usa.com
Juzo, 800 222-4999; www.juzousa.com
Medi, 76 W. Seegers Road, Arlington Heights, Ill 60005; 800-633-
    6334; www.mediusa.com
Sigvaris, PO Box 570, Branford, CT 06405; 800-322-7744;
    www.sigvaris.com

exert compression to the surface of the limb. The maximum and minimum pressures are called working and resting pressures, respectively. A nonelastic compression dressing resists stretching and exerts pressure during muscle contraction or movement. A rigid bandage has an absolute resistance against volume increase and will provide high pressure during contraction and low pressure during relaxation. A long-stretch elastic dressing changes its pressure very little during contraction and relaxation; therefore it has a high working pressure and a high resting pressure. Short-stretch material has a high working pressure and low resting pressure, which works effectively with the calf muscle pump. Long-stretch bandages can be extended up to 200%, whereas the short-stretch bandage extends from 30% to 90% [36]. When resting pressure is high for an extended period of time, arterial inflow may be compromised. Dressings with high resting pressures (long-stretch bandages and compression stockings) should be removed when the patient is not ambulating.

There are many commercially available compression systems. The oldest dressing in use for the venous ulcer is the Unna's paste boot, a rigid support dressing. A contact layer may be placed over the ulcer to prevent adherence of the dressing, or the paste bandage may be placed directly on the wound. The dressing is wrapped from below the toes to just below the knees. Extra padding may be used to absorb drainage, and the entire dressing is wrapped with an elastic bandage or wrap. The purpose of the dressing is to provide a rigid frame on the leg against which the muscle pushes during ambulation. The dressing prevents edema, and the muscle contraction squeezes the veins propelling venous blood toward the heart (Fig. 6).

When the ulcers have healed, patients should continue to wear compression stockings. The pressure prescribed should be within the 30- to 40-mm Hg range. Compression therapy is intended to prevent

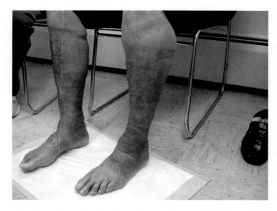

Fig. 6. A patient after the removal of a Unna boot. Brown skin pigmentation and prominent veins are characteristic changes representing chronic venous disease. Edema is reduced because the patient has been wearing a dressing.

postphlebotic syndrome and ulceration, which occurs in the lower leg; therefore, the stocking does not have to be any longer than knee-high to obtain the intended effect. Some patients, especially the elderly, find it difficult to don the tight compression stocking. Other devices that can be used in place of the stockings include rigid dressings that wrap around the leg and attach to themselves. The most important consideration when selecting a compression device is acceptance by the patient, because if it is not worn, the stocking will not work.

Surgical intervention for venous ulcers

Most venous ulcers are treated conservatively with dressings and the management of edema. There is no absolute effective surgical treatment for venous ulcers. Surgeons are reluctant to operate, creating a new wound in an area that has been difficult to heal. Some operations that have been attempted with varying results are skin grafts and free tissue flap transfer [37,38]. Subfascial endoscopic perforating vein surgery is a procedure to ligate incompetent perforator veins believed to directly contribute to venous hypertension at the ulcer site. This procedure is often combined with saphenous vein ligation and stripping. It is recommended for recalcitrant venous ulcers when incompetent perforators under the ulcer are documented by duplex scanning and Doppler ultrasonographic assessment [39,40]. One study [41] found that undergoing a saphenous vein surgical procedure was reported to have a positive effect on the quality of life for patients with CEAP class 2 to 6 disease.

Ulcers with combined causes

Approximately 25% of patients with leg ulcers for all reasons have an arterial component [42]. Patients with a nonhealing lower extremity ulcer and an ABI below 8 should be referred to a vascular surgeon to determine whether there is an underlying arterial problem that prohibits ulcer healing. These ulcers will not heal if the arterial component is not addressed. It is imperative to note that these ulcers are not just skin deep but have a complex cause and therefore require complex treatments. Making the right dressing choices, although important, is the least likely intervention to promote wound healing in these patients.

Wound treatment

Wound treatment is covered elsewhere in this issue, but there are caveats that go with vascular wounds that bear repeating. The treatment of lower extremity vascular ulcers is focused primarily on the cause of the ulcer and secondarily on the wound itself. Increasing the blood supply to the ischemic wound is critical. Patient positioning to facilitate blood flow may be of some help in arterial ulcers and is a significant part of the treatment for venous ulcers. Arterial ulcers are kept dry until revascularization is performed. If moist dressings are used, necrotic tissue in the wound can become infected. Wounds with mixed causes should be referred to a vascular specialist.

Long-term follow up

Patients with peripheral arterial or venous disease are not "cured." They must be managed throughout their lives. This requires regular preventive health care visits with a primary health care provider and routine follow-up diagnostic testing. Treatment includes risk factor management: controlling weight, smoking cessation, and drug therapy for hyperlipidemia and hypertension.

Nursing management

Although there are new modalities for identifying and treating lower extremity ulcers, revascularizing the ischemic ulcer and providing compression for the venous ulcer are still necessary. Patient education is the most important nursing intervention for lower extremity ulcers resulting from any cause. Risk factor management is the primary patient responsibility for controlling both arterial and venous disease processes and preventing further tissue deterioration. Patients who assume ownership for their own health care do better. Understanding the disease process allows patients to see the relationship of actions to outcomes. Patient education topics include disease process, medication administration, smoking cessation, nutrition, positioning, foot care, shoe wear, wound care, inspecting, moisturizing, nail trimming, and need for follow-up visits to the health care provider. These points are appropriate for patients with either venous or arterial problems. In addition, there are some things patients should know that are specific to either ischemic or venous ulcers (Table 1).

Ischemic Ulcers

Patients should be instructed to become aware of those activities that aggravate ischemia or increase the chance of injuring the extremity or the ulcer. Shoes that are too tight may create pressure points leading to soft tissue injury. Exposure to cold or continuing to smoke may cause vasoconstriction and further ischemia. Patients are taught to care for the ulcer and to monitor and report changes that occur in the ulcer and surrounding tissue. They should become familiar with signs and symptoms that represent significant progression of the disease process. Patients who have undergone bypass procedures or stent placement are taught how to monitor graft status by palpating graft and peripheral pulses (Fig. 7).

Table 1
Comparison of arterial and venous ulcer characteristics

Ulcer characteristic	Arterial	Venous
Location	Tips of toes, distal to arterial stenosis over bony prominence, metatarsals, malleoli, between toes, at pressure points	Around ankle, medial malleolus
Ulcer base	Pale, gray, yellow, no evidence of new tissue growth May be shallow or deep	Red base May be shallow or deep moist
Borders	Regular, conform to injury if ulcer was traumatic	Irregular
Drainage	Minimal	Moderate to copious
Pain	Painful (burning, throbbing, stabbing) unless neuropathy is present	Aching, stinging, burning, heaviness
Surrounding skin	Pale, dry cool, may be thin	Ruddy or with purple hue, edematous, macerated May be thick and fibrotic, oozing or crusted
Pulses	Absent or diminished	Present but may be difficult to palpate through edema

Venous Ulcers

Whatever the caregiver can do to impress on the patient the importance of compression in venous ulcer management should be done. Teaching includes information about normal venous anatomy and physiology and pathophysiology of venous disease, monitoring and recognizing potential problems, edema management, skin and nail care, and when to call the health care provider.

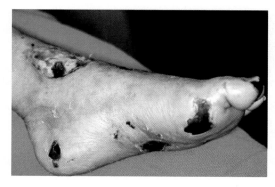

Fig. 7. An ischemic foot with chronic ulcers covered with black eschar. The ankle ulcer has a dry base, well-demarcated borders, and no drainage.

Summary

The prevalence of peripheral arterial disease in the general population is high, but the awareness of primary care providers of the disease process is low. The disease is not recognized by primary care providers [43]. Early recognition and treatment of venous diseases that progress to postphlebotic syndrome, such as after a deep vein thrombosis, will prevent venous ulcers that add considerable expense to the health care system [34]. Vascular assessment, including routine ABI measurement of patients who are in risk categories for vascular disease will identify those patients so that prevention programs can be put into place early. Major contributions to the understanding and management of leg ulcers and wound healing have been made in the last decade. However, there is still confusion as to the exact mechanism behind ulcer development and the best method to manage, cure, and prevent these ulcers has yet to be found.

References

[1] Criqui MH. Epidemiology and prognostic significance of peripheral arterial disease. In: Hirsch AT, editor. Peripheral arterial disease and intermittent claudication. The American Journal of Medicine Primary Care Series. Hillsborough (NJ): Excerpta Medica Inc; 2001. p. 5–11.

[2] Weitz JI, Byrne J, Clagett GP, et al. Diagnosis and treatment of chronic arterial insufficiency of the lower extremities: a critical review. Circulation 1996;94:3026–49.

[3] American Heart Association fact sheet. American Heart Association; 2004.

[4] Graham ID, Harrison MB, Nelson EA, et al. Prevalence of lower-limb ulceration: a systematic review of prevalence studies. Adv Skin Wound Care 2003;16:305–16.

[5] Margolis DJ, Bilker W, Santanna J, et al. Venous leg ulcer: incidence and prevalence in the elderly. J Am Acad Dermatol 2002;46:381–6.

[6] Wipke-Tevis DD, Rantz MJ, Mehr DR, et al. Prevalence, incidence, management, and predictors of venous ulcers in the long-term-care population using the MDS. Adv Skin Wound Care 2000;13:218–24.

[7] Nelzen O, Bergqvist D, Lindhagen A. The prevalence of chronic lower-limb ulceration has been underestimated: results of a validated population questionnaire. Br J Surg 1996;83: 255–8.

[8] Falanga V. Venous ulceration. J Dermatol Surg Oncol 1993;19(8):764–71.

[9] Wood CR, Margolis DJ. The cost of treating venous leg ulcer to complete healing using an occlusive dressing and a compression bandage. Wounds: A Compendium of Clinical Research and Practice 1992;4:138–41.

[10] Schonfeld WH, Villa KF, Fastenau JM, et al. An economic assessment of Apligraf (Graftskin) for the treatment of hard-to-heal venous leg ulcers. Wound Repair Regen 2000; 8:251–7.

[11] Franks PJ, McCullagh L, Moffatt CJ. Assessing quality of life in patients with chronic leg ulceration using the medical outcomes short form – 36 questionnaire. Ostomy Wound Manage 2003;49(2):26–37.

[12] Phillips TJ, Dover JS. Leg Ulcers. J Am Acad Dermatol 1991;25(6):965–89.

[13] Krasner D. Painful venous ulcers: themes and stories about living with the pain and suffering. J Wound Ostomy Continence Nurs 1998;25:158–68.

[14] Valencia IC, Falabella A, Kirstner RS, et al. Chronic venous insufficiency and venous leg ulceration. J Am Acad Dermatol 2001;44:401–21.

[15] Bogensberger G, Elgart G, Froelich CW, et al. Lipodermatosclerosis. Wounds: A Compendium of Clinical Research and Practice 1999;11(Suppl A):S2–6.
[16] Margolis DJ, Berlin JA, Strom BL. Risk factors associated with the failure of a venous leg ulcer to heal. Arch Dermatol 2000;136(3):425–6.
[17] Browse NL, Burnand KG. The cause of venous ulceration. Lancet 1982;2:243–5.
[18] Coleridge-Smith PD, Thomas P, Scurr JH, et al. Causes of venous ulceration: a new hypothesis. BMJ 1988;296:1726–7.
[19] Powell S. Contact dermatitis in patients with chronic leg ulcers. J Tissue Viability 1996;6(3):103–6.
[20] Ad Hoc Committee of the American Venous Forum. Classification and grading of chronic venous disease in the lower limbs: a consensus statement. In: Gloviczki P, Uao JST, editors. Handbook of venous disorders: guidelines of the American Venous Forum. London: Chapman & Hall; 1996. p. 652–60.
[21] Kistner RL, Eklof B, Masuda EM. Diagnosis of chronic venous disease of the lower extremities: the "CEAP" classification. Mayo Clin Proc 1996;71:338–45.
[22] Gardner AW, Womack CJ, Montgomery PS, et al. Cigarette smoking shortens the duration of daily leisure time physical activity in patient with intermittent claudication. J Cardiopulm Rehabil 1999;19(1):43–51.
[23] Whyman MR, Fowkes FG, Kerracher EM, et al. Is intermittent claudicating improved by percutaneous angioplasty: a randomized controlled trial. J Vasc Surg 1997;26:551–7.
[24] Brook RD, Weder AB, Grossman PM, et al. Management of intermittent claudication. Cardiol Clin 2002;20(4):521–34.
[25] Money SR, Herd JA, Isaacson JL, et al. Effect of cilostazol on walking distances inpatients with intermittent claudication cause by peripheral vascular disease. J Vasc Surg 1998;27(2):267–74.
[26] Beebe HG, Dawson DL, Cutler BS, et al. A new pharmacological treatment for intermittent claudication: results of a randomized, multicenter trial. Arch Intern Med 1999;27(17):2041–50.
[27] Carson SN, Overall K. Adjunctive therapy for ischemic wounds using cilostazol. Wounds 2003;15(3):77–82.
[28] Van Bemmelen PS, Weiss-Olmanni J, Ricotta JJ. Rapid intermittent compression increases skin circulation in chronically ischemic legs with infra-popliteal arterial obstruction. Vasa 2000;29(1):47–52.
[29] Banga JD, Idezerda JG, Eikelboom BC. Intermittent compression therapy in patient with leg ischemia. Presented at the 17th World Congress Meeting of the International Union of Angiology. April, 1995.
[30] Eze AR, Comerota AJ, Cisek PL, et al. Intermittent calf and foot compression increases lower extremity blood flow. Presented at the Society for Clinical Vascular Surgery's 24th Annual Symposium on Vascular Surgery. March, 1996.
[31] Vella A, Carlson L, Blier B, et al. Circulator boot therapy alters the natural history of ischemic limb ulceration. Vasc Med 2000;5:21–5.
[32] Labropoulos N, Wierks C, Suffoletto B. Intermittent pneumatic compression for the treatment of lower extremity arterial disease: a systematic review. Vasc Med 2002;7:141–8.
[33] Vogeley CL, Coeling H. Prevention of venous ulceration by use of compression after deep vein thrombosis. J Vasc Nurs 2000;18(4):123–7.
[34] Rudolph D. Standards of care for venous leg ulcers: compression therapy and moist wound healing. J Vasc Nurs 2001;19(1):20–7.
[35] Ramelet AA. Compression therapy. Dermatol Surg 2002;28(1):6–10.
[36] Hirai M. Changes of interface pressure under elastic and short-stretch bandages in posture and exercise. Phlebologie 1998;13:25–8.
[37] Steffee TJ, Caffee HH. Long term results following free tissue transfer for venous stasis ulcers. Ann Plast Surg 1998;41(2):131–7.

[38] Kumers NH, Weinzweig N, Schuler JJ. Free tissue transfer provides durable treatment for large nonhealing venous ulcers. J Vasc Surg 2000;32(5):848–54.

[39] Iafrati MD, Pare GJ, O'Donnell TF, et al. Is the nihilistic approach to surgical reduction of superficial and perforator vein incompetence for venous ulcer justified? J Vasc Surg 2002; 36(6):1167–74.

[40] Tawes RL, Barron ML, Coello AA, et al. Optimal therapy for advanced chronic venous insufficiency. J Vasc Surg 2003;37:545–51.

[41] MacKenzie RK, Lee AJ, Paisley A, et al. Patient, operative, and surgeon factors that influence the effect of superficial venous surgery on disease-specific quality of life. J Vasc Surg 2002;36(5):896–902.

[42] Treiman GS, Copland S, Mcnamara RM. Factors influencing ulcer healing in patients with combined arterial and venous insufficiency. J Vasc Surg 2001;33:1158–64.

[43] Hirsch AT, Criqui MH, Treat-Jacobson D, et al. Peripheral arterial disease detection, awareness, and treatment in primary care. JAMA 2001;286(11):1317–24.

ELSEVIER
SAUNDERS

Nurs Clin N Am 40 (2005) 411–418

NURSING
CLINICS
OF NORTH AMERICA

Index

Note: Page numbers of article titles are in **boldface** type.

0029-6465/05/$ - see front matter © 2005 Elsevier Inc. All rights reserved.
doi:10.1016/S0029-6465(05)00043-5

Changing Your Address?

Make sure your subscription changes too! When you notify us of your new address, you can help make our job easier by including an exact copy of your Clinics label number with your old address (see illustration below.) This number identifies you to our computer system and will speed the processing of your address change. Please be sure this label number accompanies your old address and your corrected address—you can send an old Clinics label with your number on it or just copy it exactly and send it to the address listed below.

We appreciate your help in our attempt to give you continuous coverage. Thank you.

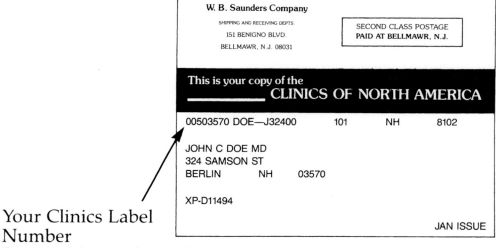

W. B. Saunders Company

SHIPPING AND RECEIVING DEPTS.
151 BENIGNO BLVD.
BELLMAWR, N.J. 08031

SECOND CLASS POSTAGE
PAID AT BELLMAWR, N.J.

This is your copy of the
_____ CLINICS OF NORTH AMERICA

00503570 DOE—J32400   101   NH   8102

JOHN C DOE MD
324 SAMSON ST
BERLIN   NH   03570

XP-D11494

JAN ISSUE

Your Clinics Label Number
Copy it exactly or send your label
along with your address to:
W.B. Saunders Company, Customer Service
Orlando, FL 32887-4800
Call Toll Free 1-800-654-2452

Please allow four to six weeks for delivery of new subscriptions and for processing address changes.